COVID-19 Lockdown

Unreported Truths Perspective

SARS-CoV-2 & COVID-19

Dr. Etch Shaheen, M.D.

Published by Knowledge is Power Publishing, part of On Call Enterprises, Inc. P.O. Box 4238, Lake Charles, Louisiana 70606.

Any information, name, phone number, physical or internet address, reference, company name or service printed in this book is this book is offered as a resource and not intended to imply agreement or endorsement by KIP Publishing, nor does KIP Publishing guarantee their accuracy or existence.

This book is intended for informative and entertainment purposes. It is not intended to serve as medical advice or any advice of any kind. If anyone has a medical condition, they should seek the advice of their physician or a qualified medical expert. No one should make any decision regarding their health, behavior, public health decisions, medical treatment, medications, or any other aspect based on what is contained in this book. The author and publisher assume no responsibility for anyone's healthcare or other matters, including but not limited to decisions related to whether to seek medical attention, what type of precautions to take, where to seek medical attention, what provider or entity to choose, what medical related decisions to make, investment decisions, or any other decisions or actions, etc. Such decisions are important, and you should consult with trusted and appropriate professionals i.e. your physician, public health officials, CDC, etc., who are experts and knowledgeable about the particulars of your specific circumstances.

ISBN 978-1-952827-10-5

Anna & Charlie

Table of Contents

Introduction

Is it possible that our schools would all close and millions of Americans would be confined to their homes? Is it possible that ordinary well-intentioned citizens are threatened with arrest or imprisonment for simply wanting to go to work? Instead of a country that values the rights of an individual, has America become a place where mayors and governors decide to become mini-dictators and order law abiding citizens to obey their self-proclaimed executive and emergency orders?

Like many others, when I first heard of some virus that was affecting Wuhan China in late December 2019 and early January of 2020, I did not pay much attention to it. Over the course of the following days and weeks, as I heard of more and more people being affected and dying, it caught my attention. As it turns out, "the original case of the novel coronavirus (that would later be officially named SARS-CoV-2) emerged on November 17, according to data from the Chinese government reviewed by South China Morning Post."[i] When I heard stories of people in the entire city of Wuhan being confined to their homes, and in some cases entrances to their homes being welded shut and armed personnel patrolling the abandoned streets, I was concerned the Chinese government was not telling the world what they may have known. I wanted to know more. Is this thing, this virus that some referred to as the Wuhan Virus or Wuhan Flu at time, as bad as it is starting to sound? Being a physician and aware of what occurred with the 1918 "Spanish Flu" Pandemic, I wondered if this new virus could be something like that. Was this being blown out of proportion so the media could pull in more viewers, or could it be some secret biologic experiment that went wrong?

While I do not consider myself a conspiracy theorist, I like to verify certain things. Especially information that is important to get right and that can have significant ramifications. I try to investigate things that do not "make sense," or seem unusual to me. In such cases, I read, speak to knowledgeable people, and try not to be naïve. I try to better educate myself. As a physician, I often look at X-rays or CT scans myself even if the radiologist has already made a reading. It is not that I do not trust their interpretation, I just feel better if I can look at the image myself and verify his report. Almost always, I discover the reading to be accurate and consistent with what I have found "clinically." i.e. what I suspect after taking a thorough history and performing a physical exam. But when the radiologist's reading of the X-ray or scan is unexpected, or does not "make sense," I make sure to review the X-ray or scan. On occasion, the report is incorrect. The radiologist may have looked at the wrong patient's scan, the medical record number may have been incorrectly entered, an old image may have been saved under the wrong patient's medical record number, the transcriptionist or transcription software, may have transcribed the report incorrectly, etc. Over the years, I have learned to trust but verify as it often helps me understand things that initially do not seem to make sense. After investigating for myself, I often discover information that helps to reconcile matters.

I understand that governments have done things that they do not announce, or people do not learn about until after the fact. I think of the Japanese government and its representatives and the "scientific experiments" they did with their prisoners of war during World War II, what the Nazi Germany did to Jews in concentration camps, and the United States government with the Tuskegee Airmen, etc. I have learned over the years to trust but verify things, especially when things seem unusual or just do not seem right. Some call this that "little voice" inside your head or "when the hair stands up on the back of your neck." Others call it that "funny feeling you get." As a physician who knows a bit about infections, viruses, "typical" symptoms and how viruses affect people, what I was seeing on TV, hearing, and reading in the media did not seem right in 2020.

I tried to rationalize. I thought, this is China, a communist country. This is the country that kills its own people and lies about it. Remember Tiananmen Square on June 3 or 4, 1989 when government troops reportedly opened fire on civilians and students who were protesting for change and tanks reportedly ran over unarmed protestors.[ii] China is the country where the government forces about a million or so Uyghur Muslims into "labor factories"[iii] to produce goods for large for profit corporations. The Chinese government has been condemned for detaining people in internment camps, which are basically prisons, where the "prisoners" are subjected to ideological, and behavioral re-education.[iv] This is the same government that arrested Dr. Li Wenliang for "spreading rumors" after he tried to warn others about this virus (SARS-CoV-2) and its dangers on social media.[v] While I thought what I was watching with the lockdown that was occurring in Wuhan China was strange, I reconciled things in my head by thinking that the Chinese government does lots of things that many would not consider kind or fair. I remember thinking to myself how lucky I was to live in the United States where something like this would never happen.

On January 21, 2020, the Center for Disease Control and Prevention (CDC) announced the first case of the coronavirus virus, the virus that causes COVID-19, in someone in the United States.[vi] [vii] The diagnosis was made in a man in Washington State who had traveled from Wuhan China. On Saturday, February 29, 2020, the CDC announced the first death in the United States attributed to "the virus that causes COVID-19."[viii]

On March 19, 2020, California Governor Gavin Newsom issued a stay at home (lockdown) order directing all residents to stay at home and "closing all businesses deemed nonessential by the state."[ix] This was the first state to issue a statewide "lockdown." By April 7, 2020, over forty (40) states and the District of Columbia had declared a stay at home or some form of restriction on its citizens.[x] During this time, I watched television and surfed the internet in amazement and disbelief. I listened to reporters, elected officials and representatives from the medical community and got that "feeling" that told me that something did not jive. I heard that "voice" that told me something is not making sense. America was being shut down. Schools and businesses were being closed by government leaders and the thriving economy that was the envy of the world and helps hundreds of millions around the world live better lives, was suddenly crippled because of the orders and actions of government leaders. At one point, "more than 41 million Americans had filed for unemployment insurance since the spread of COVID-19, according to data from the U.S. Department of Labor."[xi]

Was this "virus thing" that bad? Was there something that we are not being told or did not know? Did our leaders lose their minds and make decisions that would shut down the economy and lead to more human suffering around the world than the virus itself? Or were they getting bad information and making good decisions based on this bad information? Were they simply reacting without considering the full consequences of what they were doing? I felt as if I was watching an episode of the Twilight Zone. Perhaps worse, I felt I was in a real-life episode of the Twilight Zone. We are not in China. This is the United States of America.

Do not get me wrong, I understand this whole thing is complicated. Anyone who says otherwise does not understand the magnitude or complexity of the matter. There are health, social, economic, political, and other issues to consider. And many are intertwined i.e. economic issues significantly affect the health and well-being of people here and globally. I cannot help but wonder what our leaders were told, or believed, that led them to make the decisions they made. Their decisions impacted so many lives and will certainly lead to significant health and financial consequences. I imagine these decisions will be discussed and debated for some time. I hope we can learn from these discussions.

Because the actions of our "leaders" did not make sense to me, I decided to do what I normally do in such circumstances. I investigated for myself to learn more and find the "truth." I searched for information and data that I can look at and analyze for myself as opposed to trusting what someone reports or their interpretation of the data. I try to see if there is information that I am not aware of that may change the way I feel and make things make sense. I tried to keep an open mind and not research with the intention of proving or disproving. Instead, I wanted to find the facts and form an opinion on the matter after researching and analyzing the data. Put another way, I looked for the truth. I do try to verify what I believe I already know but remain open to learning that what I think I know now may change as I seek and learn the truth. During this journey to find the truth, I asked myself certain questions and will try to answer them for you in this book and its sequel *Lockdown 2020: Consequences & Perspective*. These questions include:

1) What is Coronavirus, where did it come from and how is it spread?
2) How can people protect themselves and lower the chances of getting infected?
3) What is the difference between masks and respirators? What protects the best? Are surgical masks effective?

Are cloth masks effective? To the person wearing the mask or others?

4) What is the difference between Coronavirus and COVID-19? What is the official name and why was it chosen?

5) How many people have caught or tested positive for coronavirus?

6) How many people have died from COVID-19? How is this number calculated? Is everyone aware the criteria for how the deaths are counted changed during the pandemic?

7) What types of tests are there for Coronavirus? How accurate are they?

8) Why were the predictions for coronavirus so wrong?

9) What are the consequences of the lockdown? Deaths? Financial? Suffering?

10) What "mistakes" or "miscues" may have been made?

11) How can we be better prepared for, or prevent, a similar pandemic in the future?

In *COVID-19 Lockdown: Unreported Truths & Perspective*, there are four chapters that will cover background information and many important and useful "fundamentals" everyone should know about SARS-CoV-2, predictions for SARS-CoV-2, diagnostic testing, and death statistics. The information is based on what facts, figures, knowledge, data, and information are known at the time this book was in manuscript form (late June to as recent as July 4, 2020).

In the next book in the series, *Lockdown 2020: Consequences and Perspective*, I will provide and discuss data illustrating the consequences of the reaction or policy response of our "leaders" to SARS-CoV-2 and COVID-19. I will show the impact upon hundreds of millions of people in the United States. The physical and mental health, child and domestic abuse, hunger, financial and personal consequences. The financial consequences that are about much more than money. The consequences impact the health of Americans, and millions around the world, perhaps even more than SARS-CoV-2 or COVID-19 impacted them. Tens of millions of people may ultimately die because of the effects that the economic downturn caused because of the policy and decisions of government leaders. Finally, I will provide some thoughts on what we have, or should have, learned and how we can do better to prevent making the same mistakes in the future.

Chapter One:

Coronavirus Fundamentals

Definition of Coronavirus

What is the Definition of coronavirus? According to Miriam-Webster, coronavirus is "any of a family (*Coronaviridae*) of large single-stranded RNA viruses that have a lipid envelope studded with club-shaped spike proteins, infect birds and many mammals including humans, and include the causative agents of Middle East Respiratory Syndrome (MERS), Severe Acute Respiratory Syndrome (SARS), and Coronavirus Disease 2019 (COVID-19)."[xii] The current coronavirus causing the pandemic (SARS-CoV-2) is not the only coronavirus. Coronaviruses are a family of viruses that can cause illnesses such as COVID-19, MERS, SARS or the common cold. The "new coronavirus" that was identified as the cause of a disease outbreak in China in 2019 is the one officially named SARS-CoV-2. The coronavirus is very small in size. It is estimated to be between "0.06 micron and 0.14 micron in diameter, averaging about 0.125 microns"[xiii] in size. As a point of reference, a human red blood cell is about 50 times larger with a diameter of about 7 microns.

Naming of SARS-CoV-2 and COVID-19

What is the official name of the virus, who named it and how was the name determined? The official name designated for this coronavirus is SARS-CoV-2 which stands for Severe Acute Respiratory Syndrome Coronavirus 2. It is not COVID-19. COVID-19 is the official name for the illness caused by SARS-CoV-2. "The Coronavirus Study Group (CSG) of the International

Committee on Taxonomy of Viruses (ICTV) named the virus SARS-CoV-2 based upon its genetic relationship to the original SARS-CoV (SARS-CoV-1) that caused an outbreak of disease in 2002-2003."[xiv] The original SARS-CoV-1 originated in Foshan, Guangdong, China, on 16 November 2002.[xv] SARS-CoV-2 has been called the Wuhan flu, or Wuhan virus, naming it after the city in China where it was first emerged. It has been called novel coronavirus. Many refer to it as the coronavirus. Some call the coronavirus virus COVID-19, but this is technically incorrect. COVID-19 is not the name of the virus itself.

It would seem less confusing and make sense to call the virus the Wuhan virus instead of a combination of letters and numbers. This has been done with many other viruses that have been named after where they originated or were first discovered to cause infections i.e. Lyme disease (Lyme Connecticut)[xvi], "West Nile virus that emerged in the West Nile district of Northern Uganda,"[xvii] "MERS caused by a virus first identified in 2012"[xviii] named after the Middle East where it is believed to have begun, Coxsackie virus after Coxsackie, New York.[xix] Etc. However, in recent years, it was decided to avoid names that that may lead to negative or "inflammatory connotations with people and places."[xx] Some allege that hate speech has been directed at Chinese people and it is thought to occur because the virus was referred to by a name associated with a Chinese geographic origin. In my opinion such unacceptable behavior has less to do with a name and more likely due to underlying ignorance and prejudice. I am not sure simply changing the way a virus is named will solve this problem, but that is for another conversation. Ironically, the WHO often refers to the coronavirus (SAR-CoV-2) incorrectly. It calls it COVID-19, which is technically not the name of the virus, but instead the name of the disease caused by SARS-CoV-2. This creates confusion and may cause unnecessary fear within the public as COVID-19 implies the disease and a worse prognosis. Some believe the WHO does this to avoid confusion with the original coronavirus of 2002 (SARS-CoV-1). Perhaps the confusion could be avoided if we went back to the old way of naming illnesses i.e. after where they first affected people or were first identified.

Because of the importance of knowing the distinction, I will mention again that SARS-CoV-2 is the name of the <u>virus</u> and COVID-19 is the name of the <u>illness</u> caused by the virus. They are not the same thing. For clarification and discussion throughout this entire book, COVID-19 refers to the illness caused by SARS-CoV-2. If someone has, or shows, no signs of illness, these persons are not considered to have illness or COVID-19, even if they test positive for SARS-CoV-2; testing positive does not qualify as illness. This is reasonable since the definition given to COVID-19 is the illness caused by SARS-CoV-2. Many would agree that no symptoms in, and no known personal consequences to, someone infected by SARS-CoV-2 constitutes as no "illness," and therefore no COVID-19 diagnosis. If this is not the case, the WHO, CDC, media, and others have not done a poor job at communicating the COVID-19 illness often has no symptoms or what many would consider as an illness. Unfortunately, many reporters, politicians, medical personnel, and individuals use the two interchangeably which is wrong and can lead to misunderstandings and incorrect conclusions. If you hear of an increase in the number of cases being reported, that simply means more people have tested positive. Most people diagnosed with coronavirus, do not get COVID-19. They do not get "sick" or "ill" (have no illness), do not require hospitalization, and do not die. If the number of "new cases" are misunderstood as being COVID-19, that would imply that those people are sick, symptomatic, and less likely to have full recoveries when in fact that is not the case.

Of those who test positive, many would not know, or suspect, that they have coronavirus if the test was not done. So, whenever you hear a statistic or someone speaking, be sure to ask if they are referring to the virus (coronavirus) or the illness, Coronavirus Disease 2019 (COVID-19). If they do not know the difference, I am not sure how much credence I would give to the information and figures they are providing. This is not to say that there is no risk to coronavirus, it is just to give some perspective.

Origin of the SARS-CoV-2 virus

It is believed that humans first contracted the virus at a wet market in Wuhan China.[xxi] Wet markets are markets where many animals are butchered and sold. These markets butcher and sell things that would disgust many people including domesticated dogs, rats, bats, snakes, wolf cubs, etc. Wet markets are called such because the floors, tables and stalls are wet from melting ice and being sprayed and watered down, often mixing with blood and bodily fluid. The first SARS, that occurred in 2002-2003, caused by SARS-CoV-1 also first infected people in China and is thought to have come from bats.[xxii]

How is SARS-CoV-2 spread?

We still are not 100% sure but it is believed that it was initially spread from animal source to a human in Wuhan China. The virus has spread significantly since December 2019 and the CDC indicated that it is mainly through human to human transmission.[xxiii] Unfortunately, the World Health Organization (WHO) sent a tweet on January 14, 2020 and "cited Chinese health officials who claimed there had been no human transmissions of the novel coronavirus within the country yet."[xxiv] According to one reporter, this is that infamous tweet that was sent by the WHO: "Preliminary investigations conducted by the Chinese authorities have found no clear evidence of human-to-human transmission of the novel #coronavirus (2019-nCoV) identified in #Wuhan, #China,"[xxv] This inaccurate statement may have contributed to a false sense of security, a lack of urgency and the loss of many human lives. Had the WHO communicated on January 14, 2020 that the virus was very contagious and spread via human to human contact, it is possible that measures could have been implemented that impeded the spread and saved hundreds of thousands of lives worldwide. Table 1 shows various ways that human to human spread may occur.

Table 1

According to WebMD.com, the human to human spread is thought to occur in the following ways:[xxvi]

Droplets. When an infected person coughs, sneezes, or talks, droplets with the virus fly into the air from their nose or mouth. Anyone who is within 6 feet of that person can breathe those droplets into their lungs.
Aerosolized transmission. Research shows that the virus can live in the air for up to 3 hours. When you breathe air that has the virus floating in it, it gets into your lungs.
Surface transmission. Another way to catch the new coronavirus is when you touch surfaces that someone who has the virus has coughed or sneezed on. You may touch a countertop or doorknob that's contaminated and then touch your nose, mouth, or eyes. The virus can live on surfaces like plastic and stainless steel for 2 to 3 days. To stop it, clean and disinfect all counters, knobs, and other surfaces you and your family touch several times a day.
Fecal-oral. Studies also suggest that virus particles can be found in infected people's poop. But experts aren't sure whether the infection can spread through contact with an infected person's

> stool. If that person uses the bathroom and doesn't wash their hands, they could infect things and people that they touch.

Risk Factors for Worse Outcomes

There are certain medical conditions or underlying factors that puts someone at a higher risk of becoming severely ill i.e. developing COVID-19 or dying from the SARS-CoV-2. These include:[xxvii]

- Age older than 65 years of age
- Chronic kidney disease
- COPD (chronic obstructive pulmonary disease)
- Immunocompromised state (weakened immune system) from solid organ transplant
- Obesity (body mass index [BMI] of 30 or higher)
- Serious heart conditions, such as heart failure, coronary artery disease, or cardiomyopathies
- Sickle cell disease
- Type 2 diabetes mellitus

Infection Avoidance

Common sense and good judgment. People should try to avoid exposure to the coronavirus. Within reason, this includes avoiding sick individuals, common sense social distancing (6 feet apart) from others that may be infected (symptomatic and asymptomatic carriers), frequent hand washing with soap and water for at least 20-30 seconds, using hand sanitizer with a minimum alcohol concentration of 60% or greater, washing / disinfecting of surfaces i.e. countertops, doorknobs, railings, etc., wearing of face shields and face masks particularly when one may not be able to maintain proper distancing from others that may be infected (sick or asymptomatic). This is for the average person not at extra risk. Of course, anyone in the healthcare industry or exposed to known infected individuals will need special, or more protective equipment. I.e. respirators, face shields, enclosed suits, etc.

Personal Protection Equipment (PPE) is something few in the general public ever heard of before the coronavirus pandemic, but it is a common term today. As its name implies, it refers to the equipment one uses to protect themselves. In the broad sense, it can protect the person wearing it from chemicals, electricity, heat, biological material, particles etc. During the coronavirus pandemic, PPE typically refers to the protection equipment to protect against the coronavirus. For healthcare workers, that would be eye protection/shielding, respiratory i.e. N95 respirators, closed breathing apparatus, etc., gowns, gloves, etc. For you going to the grocery store, a mask and safe practices may be enough. One should avoid sick individuals, avoid touching one's face i.e. mouth, eyes, nose. One should wear gloves or wash hands immediately after leaving or use a hand sanitizer as soon as you get into your car in case a surface was touched that may have been contaminated. While this may seem excessive, it is something that we probably should have always been doing.

Masks and Respirators

You may hear various terms used such respirators, N95 respirators, surgical masks, and cloth masks. Table 2 points out some of the differences between respirators and masks.

Table 2

Respirators versus Masks

RESPIRATORS	MASKS
*Respirators seal tightly to the face **Should properly fit different face sizes and features	*Surgical masks fit more loosely

Includes specialized filter media	Typically, does not include specialized filter media
*Protects the wearer against potentially hazardous particles **Designed to filter out droplet nuclei from being inhaled by the health-care worker and other individuals	*Primarily made to keep particles breathed out by the wearer – for example, saliva or mucus **Designed to stop droplet nuclei from being spread (exhaled) by the patient or wearer
*N95, N99, N100	*Surgical masks, cloth masks
Should be worn by the heath-care worker, **NOT be worn by the patient	**Should be worn by the patient, **NOT** be worn by the health-care worker.

*Per 3M[xxviii]
**Per CDC website[xxix]

We often hear about or see N95 "masks." Technically, N95 masks are not masks; they are respirators. Respirators fit tightly and are meant to filter. They should be called N95 respirators. According to OSHA:

> "These are filtering facepiece half-mask respirators, sometimes referred to as N95s. A filtering facepiece respirator covers the nose and mouth, and is a tight-fitting, air-purifying respirator in which the whole facepiece functions as the filter. Filtering facepieces may or may not have an exhalation valve to help exhaled breath exit the facepiece. They need to be fit tested unless you are wearing them under voluntary use conditions. Filtering facepiece respirators filter out particles and do *not* protect against non-particulate hazards such as gases or vapors."[xxx]

The number and letter of respirators have specific meaning.

The letter (first part of the filter's classification) "uses letters i.e. N, R, or P, to indicate the filter's ability to function when exposed to oils." "N" means **N**ot resistant to oil; "R" means somewhat **R**esistant to oil; and "P" means strongly resistant to oil, or oil-**P**roof."[xxxi]

The number represents the efficiency rating of the respirator. According to the Canadian Centre for Occupational Health and Safety (CCOHS):

> "Respirator filters that collect at least 95% of the challenge aerosol are given a 95 rating. Those filters that collect at least 99% receive a "99" rating. And those that collect at least 99.97% (essentially 100%) receive a "100" rating."[xxxii]

According to Virginia Polytechnic Institute and State University (Virginia Tech), the efficiency rating "shows how efficient the respirator's filter capacity is expected to be against particles that are at least 0.3 micrometers."[xxxiii] According to a USA article, someone's post was mentioned that made the "claim that even the N95 masks used by health care workers are pointless in the face of COVID-19."

What is the size of the actual coronavirus? According to abcdust.net, "virions (or "particles") of corona viruses are spherical particles between 0.06 micron and 0.14 micron in diameter, averaging about 0.125 micron, measured by electron microscope (Zhu et al, 2020),"[xxxv] or about 50 times smaller than a red blood cell. Is the claim raised in the USA article accurate? If the diameter of SARS-CoV-2 about 1/3 of the 0.3 micron size that the respirators are based, will the coronavirus go right through the respirator and infect the wearer?

This is a legitimate question but seems to have a reasonable and reassuring answer. According to Linsey Marr, a professor of civil and environmental engineering who specializes in airborne transmission of viruses at Virginia Tech, "there is never a naked virus floating in the air or released by people."[xxxvi] "The virus attaches to water droplets or aerosols (i.e. really small droplets) that are generated by breathing, talking, coughing, etc. These consist of water, mucus protein and other biological material and are all larger than 1 micron."[xxxvii] Since the masks can filter particles 0.3 microns, the 1micron or larger "virus complex," that contains the virus bound to other material, can be filtered effectively by the N95 respirator which filters particles greater than 0.3 microns in size.

According to "Lisa Brosseau, a retired professor of environmental and occupational health sciences who spent her career researching respiratory protection, 'Breathing and talking generate particles around 1 micron in size, which will be collected by N95 respirator filters with very high efficiency.'[xxxviii] This is consistent with the 0.3 micron threshold of the masks being plenty "small enough" to filter the much larger virus containing complex even if the virus is only 0.125 microns unbound.

In the early stages of the pandemic, the public was told that masks were unnecessary for the public to wear. It is possible that was what was believed by the "experts" at the time. It is also possible this was announced so the public would not suddenly go out and get the available supply or hoard masks and respirators, creating a shortage, or greater shortage, of respirators and surgical masks for those in healthcare. Of course, we now know that public health officials i.e. CDC and others, are advocating everyone "wear a mask" and some are suggesting it should be mandatory. Some consider this to be politically motivated. Others suggest mandating it would violate a person's right. I believe it makes sense to wear one. From a purely medical standpoint, I see little potential harm in wearing a mask or respirator, but this does not take into consideration an individual's rights, or the constitutionality of the matter if mandated.

Interestingly, the CDC specifically recommends that N95 respirators should not be worn by patients. I would assume, and believe I have heard, public officials do not want or recommend the public to use surgical masks or N95 respirators. From a purely medical standpoint, N95 respirators are better for people i.e. not only protect others but protect you, the wearer, much better. So, if everyone wore N95 respirators, the SARS-CoV-2 should be contained as good as or better than using cloth masks. It is thought that the public officials may be making the current recommendations to help preserve surgical masks, and especially N95 respirators, for healthcare workers or others. If there were excess N95 respirators in abundant supply and were inexpensive, would the CDC recommend against the public using them? One may agree or disagree with this, but I believe it is hard to make a good argument that wearing a N95 respirator makes the wearer worse off or exposes those around the wearer any more than a surgical mask, cloth mask or no mask at all.

A surgical mask is thought to protect those around the wearer from the person wearing the mask. There is, or may be, some protection to the wearer of the surgical mask. This is contrary to what public health officials initially told the public. Much less than with a N95 respirator, the surgical mask's fit is not as tight and does not have a rating like a respirator. The cloth masks may protect others from the wearer of the mask and there is a possibility that the cloth mask might provide some protection to the wearer. If so, it is likely to be much less than a surgical mask, and even less when compared to the N95 respirator.

But to be clear, neither the surgical mask nor cloth mask should be considered adequate protection. Neither provides enough protection to the person donning the mask. One puts themselves in danger if they rely on either to provide adequate protection. While the N95 respirator provides much better protection than either surgical or cloth masks, there is no guarantee it will prevent someone from being infected.

It is worth mentioning that if we practiced common sense and good hygiene on a regular basis along with common sense PPE i.e. washing hands regularly, cleaning surfaces, avoiding sick people, wearing gloves, masks and shields, etc., it is likely that the spread of many infections could be impeded, and we could save many lives. It is estimated that 30,000 to 50,000 persons die from influenza viral infections on average, every year in the United States.[xxxix] If we used face protection and washed hands and surfaces regularly, socially distanced, etc. many of these deaths may be prevented. If we washed our hands regularly, many cases of infections caused by contaminated foods could be avoided. I.e. food handlers should not have to be reminded to wash their hands after using the bathroom before returning to work. I am not advocating that we do all these things but from a pure medical standpoint, it is likely to be beneficial. Whether or not it is worth the inconveniences, sacrifices or potentially violating a person's right is a separate matter and would need to be considered.

Science

We often hear politicians, doctors, leaders, and scientists say things like "we have to follow the science," or we "base our decisions on science," etc. As a physician, I understand the importance of science and research, discovery, finding answers and solving problems, based on facts, without bias. This should be the goal of anyone in medicine, science, politics, business or most any other field. Unfortunately, some use the term science without appearing to understand what the term really means, only use "biased science," or ignore the limitations of the scientific findings they cite. They often ignore the science that does not support their views or opinions. Respectable scientists should not ignore facts or information even if it contradicts their hypothesis or the results they anticipate. Scientists should seek the truth.

One should also understand that science is not always right. Whether due to a flawed design of how the research was done, inaccurate data, bias of the researchers, unknown errors, incorrect assumptions that the findings apply to other circumstances when it actual does not, or many other, sometimes unpredictable reasons, science can be wrong. The hard part is we often do not know if or when it is wrong. That is why we must be open to information and findings that challenge the status quo i.e. our present understanding. By welcoming different views and considering challenges to the current science, we make sure the current science and the current beliefs are the best and most accurate as can be based on all the information and science available to us. Science, and beliefs based on science, should be able to stand up to challenge. It would be consistent with the assumption that the "current" science is the most correct it can be based on what is known at the current time. Honest and insightful scientists realize that science, and beliefs based on science, can change as we learn more and advance.

There was a time when the "great minds" of the time thought the world was flat, until it was not. As we learn more, or better studies and research is done, science often proves the previous findings of science wrong. More recently, "experts" implied or stated that the SARS-CoV-2 was not easily transmitted by human to human contact, that masks were unnecessary or did not protect the wearer. So, while we should "trust the science," we should also understand that the science can sometimes be wrong. We must be open to listening to other ideas and thoughts that may not necessarily agree with the current accepted science. We must investigate and challenge current thinking. We never know for sure if the current science is correct or will be replaced by more correct science as science evolves. Keep this in mind, particularly when some criticize others with different opinions.

During the current COVID-19 pandemic, there were two emergency physicians in Bakersfield California, Drs. Dan Erickson and Artin Massihi, who expressed their opinions on COVID-19 related matters. I do not know either of these doctors nor have any affiliation whatsoever to them. They commented that the initial projections showed millions would die and called them "woefully inaccurate."[xl] It was mentioned in an April 22, 2020 article that Dr. Erickson cited Kern County, California statistics of 340 positive COVID cases out of 5213 people being tested yielding an estimated 6.5% of the population being positive, and 33,865 COVOD cases out of a total of 280,900 tested in the entire state of California, indicating about 12% of the state population is positive for COVID-19. It is unclear from the article if when they used the term "tested positive for COVID" whether they meant simply tested positive for SARS-CoV-2 or had the illness of COVID-19 and tested positive for SARS-CoV-2. The two physicians apparently own or work at urgent care facilities in Kern County that performed testing for SARS-CoV-2 and were reported to have done over 50% of all the tests performed in their county. The two held a press conference on April 24, 2020, and provided their thoughts and opinions regarding COVID-19.[xli] "Now that we have the facts," said Dr. Erickson. "It's time to get back to work."[xlii] "Dr. Erickson asked if numbers that low necessitated people sheltering in place, shutting down medical systems and putting people out of work."[xliii]

To be transparent, I did not watch the complete press conference but did see parts of it on television and online. I was a bit surprised by the response to it. Many in the medical community criticized them. Some physicians on medical blogs called for action against the two including censoring them, reprimanding them, even suggesting threatening their medical license. Apparently, the press conference was uploaded onto YouTube by 23ABC. According to an April 30, 2020 article, "on April 27th 23ABC received an email from YouTube giving the station notification the video had been taken down, citing YouTube's "community guidelines."[xliv] According to the article, that decision is being appealed. YouTube indicated that the video was pulled because "the content contradicted the guidance of the local health authority."[xlv] Based on the response to their comments/press conference, it appears that others did not approve of, or agree with, what they said. I find the response from the medical community, the media and YouTube concerning. Perhaps we should all be alarmed by how two physicians were criticized, some may say "condemned" just because they were expressing their opinions and exercising their right to free speech.

Without getting into a long discussion about whether they have a responsibility, or obligation, to only spread the same message as government agencies, politicians or popular views, as a society, we need to take a big breath and come to our senses. It is a dangerous thing to try to silence, discredit or attack someone because they have a different opinion. If someone disagrees with you, you should not attack them especially. One would not expect this, especially in the "scientific" community. If you wish to respond, you can respond with facts or point out the issue, opinion, or fact that you disagree with. You can have a constructive discussion. I did not necessarily agree with everything these physicians may have said but I did not disagree with everything either. Instead of reflexively responding or attacking them, perhaps people should consider what was said, realize the limitations of the knowledge we know about SARS-CoV-2 and COVID-19, and the many other, and consider their information and opinion. I am not implying that anyone should accept their opinion as gospel, I am simply suggesting that perhaps we should think and question what we think we already know and what they said. By doing so, we make ourselves think and challenge information. If information is good and knowledge is sound, it should withstand challenge and be able to provide unbiased facts and data to support and prove it. If you cannot do this, then perhaps the information that you have may not be as correct as we assume it to be. This is how great minds work. Not being so arrogant to think that what we currently think or know is the only answer, or will always be the correct answer, but to consider other thoughts and ideas and put all views through rigorous challenges to prove their worth. This is how "real science" should work.

There are other arguments as to why someone should be allowed to express their opinions i.e. freedom of speech, constitutional rights, etc. but I will resist the temptation. Also, one might argue that the public should be allowed to hear different opinions and not just what their government says or approves of, or what those who agree with message the government wish to communicate. People are not stupid. In most any circumstance, people should be allowed to make free choice for themselves and be responsible and accountable for their decisions and actions.

Treatment for SARS-CoV-2 and COVID-19

For someone who has been diagnosed with the coronavirus, no treatment is typically required. Most with coronavirus have no symptoms, minor symptoms or self-limited symptoms that will get better on their own with no treatment. Symptoms may include sniffles, sore throat, fever, shortness of breath, unusual rash, loss of sense of smell or taste, headache, muscle aches, etc., a combination of any of these symptoms or no symptoms at all. People with mild or no symptoms should try to maintain good health by making sure they stay well hydrated, unless some contraindication to do so, eating a healthy diet and getting appropriate amounts of rest. These are the things people should be doing all the time regardless of whether they have SARS-CoV-2 or not. They should contact a competent and trusted medical professional and make sure they get appropriate care. Some advocate vitamin C i.e. orange juice, zinc, soup, etc. I would suggest consulting your physician and discussing your health concerns and questions. While no specific treatment i.e. medication or intervention, is often necessary, everyone should practice good hygiene by washing their hands regularly, not sharing drinking glasses, eating utensils, or exposing others, especially those at risk, to the virus. Wearing a mask helps protects others and may provide some protection to the wearer. Those especially most vulnerable i.e. elderly, obese, underlying comorbidities, need to be extra careful. Clean surfaces with appropriate disinfectants that kill the virus i.e. alcohol content > 60%. Consider wearing N95 respirators, as these provide better protection to the wearer than masks, especially when one cannot properly practice social distancing.

Those who may have more than minor symptoms i.e. fever, shortness of breath, chest pain, dizziness, headaches, unusual rashes, etc., should be seen by a medical professional. You may have COVID-19 or another condition that needs medical attention. Given the pandemic and apparent highly contagious nature of this virus, one should assume they have COVID-19 until proven otherwise. This is not to frighten you; it is a precaution. If you assume you have COVID-19, get checked by a physician and follow his or her prescribed treatment and recommendations.

If you have no symptoms and feel well, you could still be one of many who are infected without any symptoms and never develop COVID-19. If you happen to be an asymptomatic carrier, you could expose others. This is the reason to take precautions and behave as if you could have it i.e. social distancing, wear masks, hand washing, etc.

When COVID-19 first struck, there really was little in terms of treatment other than supportive care. Supportive care means providing care such as hydration/IV fluids if one is dehydrated, oxygen if one's oxygen level is lower than acceptable levels, and ventilation with a breathing machine, if necessary. We have learned from this pandemic that placing someone on positive pressure ventilation (ventilator) may harm patients. We have also discovered that having patients in the prone position (lying on one's "stomach" instead of your back) may be better than having patients positioned on their backs.

When the COVID-19 pandemic first hit "our shores," there were no medications to kill the virus or to make a significant difference in patient outcomes. As many know, antibiotics that many think of as drugs that kill infections, do little to nothing to help kill viruses. Certain antibiotics kill certain bacterial infections but do not kill viruses. That is part of the reason that doctors often tell patients, or families of patients, that they are not going to prescribe antibiotics for a sore throat, rash or fever that is believed to be from a virus or the flu. Antibiotics will not help with viral infections and can possibly cause other consequences such as contributing to the drug resistant bacteria problem in our country. It can also cause one to have side effects of the antibiotic such as nausea, vomiting, stomach pain, diarrhea, allergic reaction, and rarely an anaphylactic reaction that could be lethal.

All medications have risks. In some cases, these risks can be serious. Physicians' number one rule is to "do no harm." Before prescribing medications, responsible physicians consider the risks and benefits of medications, even when their patients request, sometimes demand, them. This is one of the reasons why physicians may not always prescribe medications, even when their patients request them. Fortunately, in most cases, there are no serious complications when medications are prescribed. In many circumstances, there is little to no benefit to taking medications. Some patients get frustrated or upset when they do not get some medication to treat whatever ailment they may have. While most people are reasonable, some believe that unless they are "treated," specifically with some pharmaceutical, they are not receiving appropriate care. Sometimes it is best to take nothing. With proper education of patients by their physicians, many are starting to understand this reality, and satisfied to be treated with observation and other non-pharmaceutical measures. Physicians must use their knowledge, available current information, and the specifics of the patient to come up with the best treatment for their patients, understanding that what is proper treatment for one person's situation or condition, may be best for another. This may be why some refer to the practice of medicine as "the art of medicine." It is not always clear cut and there is often not one right answer. This does not mean to imply that no medication will ever be indicated to prevent infection or to treat asymptomatic people or mild illnesses caused by SARS-CoV-2. Treatments and recommendations may change as we learn more. What is written here and throughout this book only applies to what I am aware of today (July 4, 2020 and before). With time, I hope, and expect, us to learn more and have more available options (pharmacologic and non-pharmacologic) that will treat or prevent COVID-19.

Medications:
Hydroxychloroquine

Hydroxychloroquine (along with a similar drug chloroquine) was initially designed to treat malaria. It was later found to be useful in the treatment of certain autoimmune disorders.[xlvi] It is not uncommon for drugs that are researched or used to treat one illness or condition to later be found to be effective against other illnesses or conditions. Hydroxychloroquine is a drug that was thought to be protective early on and many were prescribed and took it. The drug has been shown to have anti-viral properties in lab settings and thought to work by interfering with the coronavirus' ability to enter human cells and blocking the virus' ability to replicate once inside the cell.[xlvii xlviii]

President Trump was an early champion of the drug and voluntarily offered that he was taking hydroxychloroquine for prevention.[xlix] It is unclear if he was trying to avoid becoming infected with the virus or the more serious COVID-19, or both. There are many within the medical community who believe that there is benefit to the drug and prescribe it to their patients. A French study led by epidemiologist Dr. Didier Raoult reported a high success rate (98%) in patients treated with hydroxychloroquine along with the antibiotic azithromycin.[l]

However, there are also many in medical community who did not believe that hydroxychloroquine is of benefit in the treatment or prevention of COVID-19 or Coronavirus. Many in the medical community criticized the use of hydroxychloroquine and even stated that it is potentially dangerous and that benefits did not justify the risks. More studies were done. Two studies published in the BMJ did not support continued use of hydroxychloroquine.[li] The Lancet, what many consider a reputable medical journal, published a study in May 2020 that "found no benefit to the drug-and suggested its use may even increase the risk of death."[lii] Some may have believed the findings, while others may have felt there may have been an ulterior or political motive behind the findings. The study was later called into question. The Lancet retracted the study about two weeks later because of "potential flaws in the research data."[liii] [liv] Researchers from Brigham and Women's Hospital in Boston had worked with and apparently relied upon data and analysis that was conducted by a healthcare analytics company called Surgisphere Corporation. The study authors pointed out in their retraction that several concerns were raised in respect to the data and analysis.[lv] This same article cites one expert as stating "a first year statistics major could tell you about the major flaws in the design of the analysis."[lvi] What do we take from this? The study is not something we should rely on. It was flawed, potentially biased or possibly even corrupt. It does not necessarily mean hydroxychloroquine is helpful or harmful. It means the authors of the study were not able to verify the data was accurate. Without accurate data, it is hard to make certain conclusions with any degree of confidence and should not sway you one way or another.

Just prior to submitting this book's manuscript to be published, a study that was published on July 2, 2020, by Henry Ford Medical Center announced hydroxychloroquine demonstrated benefit.

> "In a large-scale retrospective analysis of 2,541 patients hospitalized between March 10 and May 2, 2020 across

the system's six hospitals, the study found 13% of those treated with hydroxychloroquine alone died compared to 26.4% not treated with hydroxychloroquine. None of the patients had documented serious heart abnormalities; however, patients were monitored for a heart condition routinely pointed to as a reason to avoid the drug as a treatment for COVID-19. The study was published today in the International Journal of Infectious Diseases, the peer-reviewed, open-access online publication of the International Society of Infectious Diseases (ISID.org)."[lvii]

While everything about this study has not been completely reviewed due to submission deadlines and one must be cautious not to rely on any one study, the preliminary results are encouraging. It is also reassuring that the Henry Ford study was peer-reviewed. It appears that only hospitalized patients were enrolled in this study. If mortality can be reduced by 50% or more by using hydroxychloroquine, as the study appears to indicate, this would be significant. Hopefully, we will learn more and other centers will also conduct studies using hydroxychloroquine and we can see if they reach the same or similar results.

In March 2020, the Food and Drug Administration (FDA) granted emergency use authorization (EUA) for hydroxychloroquine in the treatment of COVID-19 patients. This EUA allows unapproved medical products or unapproved uses of approved medical products to be used in public health emergencies.[lviii]

Remdesivir

An investigational anti-viral medication manufactured by Gilead is recommended for use, by "the COVID-19 Treatment

Guidelines Panel, in hospitalized patients who require oxygen and in patients who are on mechanical ventilation (ventilators) or require extracorporeal membrane oxygenation (ECMO)."[lix] It is not recommended for use in patients with mild to moderate COVID-19. The medicine is given intravascularly (IV) and is reported to shorten the time to recovery for severely ill hospitalized patients from 15 days to 11 day (31%).[lx][lxi] One study in April showed that remdesivir had 'no clinical benefit.'[lxii] As of June 27, 2020, I am unaware of any scientific study that claims remdesivir decreases mortality or any other antivirals that have been shown to be effective against COVID-19 and FDA approved for that purpose

Tamiflu

A medication used to treat Influenza A and B ("the flu"), is "not indicated for the prevention or treatment of SARS-CoV-2 infection."[lxiii] Tamiflu is being tested in clinical trials in conjunction with other treatments, to find out if it works to reduce length of illness, complications and the rate of death in COVID-19 patients.[lxiv]

Dexamethasone

This is a corticosteroid anti-inflammatory medication (steroid) that has been around for a long time and used for a variety of medical conditions including allergic reactions, asthma, chronic obstructive pulmonary disease (COPD), edema (swelling) in the brain associated with masses, arthritis, inflammatory conditions, etc.

In a study done in England and led by the University of Oxford, dexamethasone reduced death by 35% in patients on ventilators and by 20% in patients who required supplemental oxygen.[lxv] [lxvi] The mean age of participants in this study was 66.1 years and over half had one or more major comorbidity.[lxvii] There was no benefit reported for dexamethasone in less ill patients. The study researchers point out that dexamethasone would prevent 1 out of every 8 deaths in patients treated who required mechanical ventilation (on ventilators) and prevent 1 out of every 25 deaths in patients requiring supplemental oxygen.[lxviii] The medication was given either given orally or via IV. "Dexamethasone is the first and only drug that has made a significant difference to patient mortality for COVID-19"[lxix] according to Nick Cammath, COVID-19 Therapeutic Accelerator Lead at the Wellcome Trust health charity. A similar statement was made by Peter Horsby, a professor of Infectious Diseases in the Nuffield Department of Medicine, University of Oxford who stated "dexamethasone is the first drug to be shown to improve survival in COVID-19. This is an extremely welcome result."[lxx]

Health policy expert at Memorial Sloan-Kettering Cancer Center in New York, Dr. Peter Bach, points out that 41% of patients on ventilators, and 25% of patients on oxygen alone died in the study. He adds that "the mortality rate seems to be way higher than in the US."[lxxi]

Another author wrote that it is likely that the beneficial effect of corticosteroids in severe viral respiratory infections is dependent on using the right dose, at the right time, in the right patient."[lxxii] This is an interesting point as the WHO and others advise against using steroids early in the course of illness because doing so could impede clearing the virus. Yet the Oxford study seems indicates that using steroids in severely ill patients seems to decrease the chance of death.

According to Dr. Anthony Fauci, who has served as Director of the National Institute of Allergy and Infectious Diseases for over

30 years and became a household name during the COVID-19 pandemic,

> "Early in you're fighting the virus and you want your immune system to be as intact as possible" but in the advanced state of COVID-19, the battle against the virus causes so much inflammation that it "is hurting you more than helping you."[lxxiii]

This would reconcile the WHO's recommendations for not using steroids early in the disease and the Oxford study's finding that steroids are beneficial with severely ill patients with COVID-19.

Make no mistake, the Oxford study findings are encouraging. It appears dexamethasone helps and if so, that is great news. But we must also be cautious, it is one study. It has yet to be peer reviewed and the patient population and the factors affecting them in that study may not apply to patients elsewhere. The future will tell if others can duplicate the Oxford study findings or demonstrate the benefits of steroids. In addition, even if it works as well as the Oxford study reports, it is neither a cure nor does it save every patient. Many patients still died. Twenty-eight percent (28%) of patients on ventilators and twenty percent (20%) of patients who required oxygen still died, even with dexamethasone. The point: COVID-19, particularly when severe, is bad and kills people.

Anticoagulants

The medical community has discovered that many with COVID-19 seem to be developing a thrombotic state. In plain English, COVID-19 patients seem to be more susceptible to forming blood clots and poses even more danger to these patients. According to Dr. Behnood Bikdeli, MD, MS, a cardiovascular medicine fellow at Columbia University Irving Medical Center (CUIMC) and a specialist in thrombosis, "clotting is causing damage to other organs, and in my experience, it's above and beyond what we've seen in other acutely ill patients."[lxxiv] According to a Columbia University April 30, 2020 article, "blood clots can travel to the brain to cause strokes, the heart to cause heart attacks, and the lung to cause pulmonary embolisms, but physicians also report clot-related damage in other organs and in the lower legs of COVID-19 patients."[lxxv] Doctors have reported odd rashes and unusual coloring of the fingers and toes of some patients that could be caused by small thrombi (clots). Some experts advocate administering blood thinners to COVID-19 patients similar to what other non-COVID-19 patients receive, others believe that COVID-19 patients should be anti-coagulated more aggressively. There is a clinical study being performed at CUIMC to evaluate anti-coagulants in critical COVID-19 patients in the intensive care unit (ICU) and hospital.

Antibiotics

As previously mentioned, antibiotics have little to role in treating viruses. However, antibiotics are sometimes used in patients infected with viruses that are suspected of also having bacterial infections. There are patients that have viral infections, who's immune system may be weakened and then get a secondary bacterial infection. In these cases, it is perfectly reasonable to treat with appropriate antibiotics. There are occasions when a treating physician cannot be sure if an infection is bacterial or viral. In these cases, an antibiotic or combination of antibiotics may be used depending on the circumstances of the patient. For example, if the patient is healthy, does not appear ill, and simply has a sore throat with a normal appearing throat on exam and/or a negative

Streptococcal screening of the throat, that person will likely not be prescribed antibiotics. Yet a patient who appears ill, may have underlying medical health problems and be at risk for death or serious illness may be given antibiotics if the physician cannot be sure if the patient has a viral or bacterial infection. The reasoning is that there is less room for error and when one considers the risks vs. rewards, it is not unreasonable to try antibiotics in such cases, "just in case" there may be a dangerous bacterial infection present.

As of June 28, 2020, it appears that only dexamethasone shows a significant reduction in deaths in those severely ill enough to require oxygen or on ventilators. Remdesivir may have some benefit in shortening hospitalization of severely ill patients. That does not mean other medications are not effective, these medications will not be found to be more effective (or less), or that physicians and their patients should not be allowed to use medications that may be beneficial to the patient depending on the circumstances. With time, we often learn more and further treatments are discovered or created. One may say this is why we say that doctors "practice" medicine as we would be foolish to think that physicians know something so well that we cannot learn more or get better.

*Update, as of July 3, 2020, dexamethasone may no longer be the "only medication" that can significantly reduce mortality that we are aware. Hydroxychloroquine may also reduce mortality, as discussed above and according to the Henry Ford Health System article dated July 2, 2020. Hydroxychloroquine may help even more than dexamethasone in hospitalized or "sick" patients. Given the news that became public right before *COVID-19 Lockdown: Unreported Truths & Perspective* was to be sent for publishing, I have not had the opportunity to fully investigate the study but wanted to make sure it was mentioned. We do not know all the answers and I imagine many will have questions and further work needs to be done but it is encouraging. It is hoped that researchers will look into the benefits of one versus the other, if a combination of the two may be even more effective, if certain patients benefit from one over the other, or a combination of one, etc. Time will tell.

Chapter 2:
Predictions

Being able to accurately predict things is important so one can plan accordingly. Meteorologists try to predict the weather and we use this information to help us decide what to wear, or whether to take an umbrella with us. The ability to make accurate predictions is useful with viruses and other infectious diseases as well. To be able to make more accurate predictions for SARS-CoV-2, it is important to understand it. Important factors to know are:

- How dangerous is it if someone contracts it?
- How contagious is it?
- How is it spread?
- How many people currently have it?
- How many people are likely to contract it?
- How many people are likely to get sick from it?
- Of those who get sick, what amount and level of care and resources will they need?
- How likely are you to die from it?
- Once infected and recovered, is there immunity from future infections?
- How does it compare to other things that cause death?
- How many people will die from it?
- What options are there, and what are the benefits and consequences of each?

Knowing the answers to these and other questions can help guide public policy, determine what resources may be necessary, allow medical personnel and other agencies to prepare and to help communicate accurate and useful information to the public to help them take appropriate precautions and avoid unnecessary fear and panic.

Prediction Terms:
Actual Cases

Actual cases and confirmed cases can be different, vastly different. The number of actual cases of something may be difficult to know. It attempts to predict whether people have an illness without actually testing every person. So, one must rely on certain assumptions and estimates. We often know the confirmed cases. These are the people that you test. These are not projections or estimates based on data from others but rather specific to people who the actual data comes from. The results are either positive or negative. The patients either recover or die. Confirmed cases usually make up a portion of the real number of cases that exist. We may not know the number of people who may be infected but not tested or reported, number of people currently hospitalized who we do not know yet if they will recover or die. Actual cases may sometimes be based on closed cases i.e. people who have been hospitalized and already discharged or died.[lxxvii] Keep in mind, whenever estimates are made, there is a greater chance of error. Sometimes these errors can be significant. When calculating actual cases, various factors are taken into consideration and can be influenced by many factors. Actual case predictions are specific to a certain geographic location or a specific population.

An example is New York City. According to a May 14, 2020 article, the number of confirmed cases was reported as 166,883 in NYC. These patients were tested and tested positive. When New York State conducted an antibody study, it estimated 12.3% of the population of the state of New York was positive for antibodies to SARS-CoV-2 as of May 1, 2020. The antibody testing results estimated that 19.9% of the population of New York City had COVID-19 antibodies. This implies that 12.3% of the state and 19.9% of New York City are, or had been, infected by SARS-CoV-2. If one applies the SARS-CoV-2 "infection rate" or "prevalence" of 19.9% for New York City to population of New York City (8,398,748), the number of estimated "actual cases" that exist would be about 1,671,350. This actual case number is an estimate. We cannot know for sure the number of "real" cases without testing every single person i.e. testing 8,398,748 people in NYC. This actual case number is slightly over 10 times more than the 166,883 confirmed cases for NYC at the time. This is a significant difference, a factor of over 10.

Actual Cases (estimate) = prevalence in sample population X population of larger population

Estimated Actual number of SARS-CoV-2 in NYC= 19.9% X 8,398,748=1,671,350

One cannot extrapolate these findings to other locations and assume they apply. Also, we assume that those who were tested in the study are an accurate representation of the entire population they are trying to apply the study findings to. One must understand these are estimates and can be wrong, but the information can be valuable.

It appears that the CDC measurement of actual deaths in New York City is not what some may consider a reliable, or an exact, reflection of definite deaths, definitely caused by COVID-19 as follows:

Actual Deaths=Confirmed Deaths + Probable Deaths + Excess Deaths

Confirmed Cases

This may apply to actual cases and not projections or estimates. Yet, the number will depend of the definition assigned to this term. Initially, confirmed cases of death from COVID-19 required death and a positive test for SARS-CoV-2. It had specific criteria that is thought to include a human and non-human element (positive lab test). The person who died had to test positive and the cause of death determined to be from SARS-CoV-2 by someone, assumed to be a physician. This is presumed as it is difficult to know for sure. We do not know if only a positive test qualified as a COVID-19 related death even if the likely cause was from something else i.e. motor vehicle accident, fatal gunshot wound, heart attack, etc. We do know the initial criteria was changed after the fact (deaths that already occurred and identified with causes of death) causing the existing death counts assigned to COVID-19 to be replaced with dramatically higher counts. Lab test confirmation was no longer required, and the diagnosis could be 100% subjective i.e. probable cause of death. One might wonder if "confirmed cases" is an accurate count of actual cases of COVID-19 deaths.

Excess Deaths

'The total number of excess deaths in each jurisdiction was calculated by summing excess deaths in each week, from February 1, 2020 to present and the total number of excess deaths for the US overall was computed as a sum of jurisdiction-specific numbers of excess deaths (with negative values set to zero)." [lxxviii] According to the CDC, excess deaths is "the difference between the observed numbers of deaths in specific time periods and expected number of deaths in the same time periods." [lxxix] In plain language, if the number of observed deaths is above the expected number of deaths, the difference is called "excess deaths." This expected number is predicted by calculating the average number of deaths in that period i.e. a specific week of the year, from previous years.

**Excess Deaths* = Observed deaths in specific time period −
Expected # of deaths in same time period**

*CDC does not count negative numbers. If the number is less than zero, CDC uses zero in its calculations.

Mortality Rate

"Mortality rate, or death rate, is a measure of the number of deaths in a particular population. Mortality rate may be expressed in units of deaths per 1,000 individuals per year, per 100,000 individuals (particularly when the incidence is low) etc.; thus, a mortality rate of 9.5 (out of 1,000) in a population of 1,000 would mean 9.5 deaths per year in that entire population."[lxxx] In order to calculate this, one must know the total number in the population being measured and the total number of deaths within that population. If one is trying to calculate the mortality rate from a specific cause, i.e. COVID-19, one would have to know the population size, and the number of deaths from that specific cause.

**Mortality Rate = # of deaths within that population/# in that
population (infected and uninfected)**

For example. If 500 people die in a year in a state, from a specific cause, with a state population of 20,000,000, the mortality rate from that specific cause is calculated as follows:

Mortality rate is 500/20,000,000= 0.000025 or 0.0025% or 1 in 40,000, or 2.5 per 100,000 people

Using the total COVID-19 (SARS-CoV-19) death figure from the CDC on June 28, 2020 for June 27, 2020, of 125,484 and an estimated US population of 328,000,000, the current **mortality rate in the United States** from SARS-CoV-2 as of June 27, 2020 would be 1 in about 2614 or 0.038%

0.038% is the current mortality rate of SARS-CoV-2 for the general population of the United States as of, or about, June 27, 2020.

125,484/328,000,000=0.00038 (0.038%), or approximately 1 in 2613.88, or 38.3 per 100,000 people

In the case of **New York City, the Mortality rate is:**

23,430/8,398,748=0.00278 (0.28%) or about 1 in 358 people, or 279 per 100,000 people

0.28% is the approximate current mortality rate in New York City as of approximately May 1, 2020 (this assumes the more liberal number of deaths. If one uses only the confirmed cases at that time, if we only calculate using confirmed cases of 13,156, as opposed to 23,430, the mortality rate in New York City as of about May 1, 2020 would be 0.001566 or 0.16%, or about 1 in 638.6 people, or 156.6 people per 100,000 population.

Infection Fatality Rate (IFR)

Infection Fatality Rate is percentage of the people who become infected that die. It is calculated by dividing the number of deaths because of the infection by the total number of those who are infected. Unless everyone in a population is tested and the tests are 100% accurate, this will not be 100% accurate and there is some estimation that is often used.

Infection Fatality Rate = # Deaths / # of Total in population that are infected

Because we often do not know the "True" or real numbers of deaths or those infected, we use estimates i.e. "actual" deaths and total infected in entire population (unless everyone has been tested) One such formula is:

Infection Fatality Rate (IFR) = Actual Deaths / Total # Infected by Virus

Applying the figures that we used for New York City, the numbers are plugged in:

*Infection Fatality Rate = *23,430 / 1,671,350 =0.0140=1.4% or 1 in 71.33 people

**Infection Fatality Rate = **13,156 / 1,671,350 =0.00787=0.8% or 1 in 127.04 people

*Using CDC figures of Confirmed Cases + Probable Cases + Excess Deaths
**Using Confirmed Death cases only
The Total Infected by SARS-CoV-2 was estimated by applying the percentage of people who tested positive for SARS-CoV-2 antibodies in a sampling of people in New York City (19.9% had antibodies) multiplied by the population of New York City.
~The Infection Fatality Rate for the 1918-1919 Spanish Flu caused by the H1N1 virus is thought to have been 10%

While it is easy to criticize those responsible for public health i.e. public health officials, researchers, physicians, those in academics, one must consider that determining these factors can often be challenging. When there is an illness that is "new" and we do not have too much information about, it can sometime be difficult to be able to accurately predict all the things that are important to know.

More importantly, accurate information is critical to make accurate predictions. One must apply reasonable assumptions and common sense. If the data is accurate, assumptions are good and reasonable predicting methods are applied, using common sense, and adjusting for reasonable factors, a fairly accurate prediction can be made. This does not guarantee that the predictions will come to fruition or be 100% accurate but the predictions are more likely to be accurate. Many sports fans will understand this concept. Think of the sports handicappers that predict the outcomes of sporting events and the point spreads of games. They take into account many factors that affect a game such as the teams, the players, the location of the game, injuries, recent performance, playoff eligibility at stake, etc. and then make predictions on the outcome of the games. They are not always right and sometimes can be way off, but it is amazing how often they are correct. When predicting a virus, it is often much more challenging. There are many unknowns and the characteristics of the next one may be different than previous one.

I have great respect for researchers and those who make predictions who are honest, have integrity and a genuine desire to provide unbiased predictions based on the information available, application of acceptable and reliable prediction tools, and are introspective and critical of the predictions they make, clearly state the likelihood of the predictions being accurate, and apply good judgment and common sense. If predictions come from researchers who apply these standards, it may not be perfect, but it is likely as valuable and useful as one can get. Because the person who gets the prediction can base their decision knowing the limitations and the "magnitude" of those limitations.

Having said that, it is reasonable for some to criticize the predictions that were made with SARS-CoV-2. One prediction that may have caused a great deal of concern and led to aggressive measures by our elected officials is from the Imperial College of London. On March 26, 2020 it stated: "We estimate that in the absence of interventions, COVID-19 would have resulted in 7.0 billion infections and 40 million deaths globally this year."[lxxxi] The study reports that their estimates were based on "data from China and high-income countries" and admits that they did not take into consideration "the wider social and economic costs of suppression, which will be high and may be disproportionately so in lower income settings."[lxxxii] Interestingly, the article does not discuss the health risks or cost of human lives that may be lost from suppression (shelter in place, lock downs, etc.).

In a Forbes article, it was reported that "Dr. Birx stated that the team advising the President on COVID-19 had reviewed 12 different models, from institutions such as Imperial College of London and Columbia University. The models predicted a range of deaths between 1.6 and 2.2 million if the country took no containment measures, with at least half the country eventually becoming infected." [lxxxiii] Dr. Deborah Birx is the Coronavirus Response Coordinator for the White House. It was also reported that the University of Washington's Institute for Health Metrics and Evaluation (IHME) had similar finding.[lxxxiv] With predictions such as this, if policy makers were informed of these predictions by the team advising them and believed them, one can understand why they may have panicked and locked down the country. One can understand why many countries locked their countries.

A couple things to wonder and ask of our "leaders" is did you base your decisions on these predictions? If so, did you confirm or have other qualified, respected, and trusted experts independently review this data and perform their own predictions to compare? Did they also weigh in the consequences of locking down their populations? A couple points here. Often researchers or those who make predictions often use disclaimers that they do not consider other factors i.e. social and economic in Imperial College of London predictions, and do not specifically show prediction of human lives that will be lost because of the "suppression" and the consequences of it. The second point is that leaders ultimately are responsible for policy and should be held accountable without complete immunity. They should not be able to hide behind what others predict and have immunity from their decisions. Yes, they should consult experts from many areas, but these experts often only consider the effects regarding their area of expertise. They do not weigh the magnitude or the effect of their suggestions or recommendations on other areas and sometimes not on their own area. So, it is the responsibility and obligation of the policy makers to weigh the risks and benefits of all factors and make their decision. Their decision should not be political or based on ulterior motives but based on what is best for the country (or specific population in the area that they represent). While this is a great responsibility, it is part of the privilege of leadership and must be accepted without dilution of their responsibility and/or liability.

Some suggestions to help clear up confusion and help make predictions more useful to those who rely on them may be to:

- Clearly indicate when you do not know something that is relevant and that would be useful for your audience to know. If you do not know, or there is insufficient data or evidence to make an accurate prediction, say so. There is nothing wrong with saying we do not know or cannot make a prediction worthy of consideration. Doing so, should make whatever predictions you do make more credible.

- Clearly indicate the likelihood of the accuracy of the predictions. Tell the public "we estimate this but only with a 20% confidence interval" or "we are 95% sure it will be at least this bad, 50% sure that it will be this bad, and there is a 5% it will be this bad or worse." Give degrees of certainty for different degrees of seriousness [the number affected or how badly they will be affected i.e. require intensive care unit (ICU), or ventilators or will die]. This would be much more useful to those who make policy and to the public to reach their own conclusions.
- Clearly indicate the factors that you used that led to the predictions being that "bad." For example, indicate that on average for every 1 person who has it, we assume they are likely to infect another 2.5 people, or 8 people, etc. This may be considered an "exacerbating factor."
- Clearly indicate what the factors that make the predictions not so bad i.e. virus does not seem to be serious, create the need for hospitalization or cause death in anyone underage X. For example, even though it spread particularly badly in this population, that population was malnourished and had underlying conditions that are not present in other populations. Some may call this explaining "mitigating factors" for spread.
- Avoid vague statement that cannot be substantiated i.e. "in the absence of interventions." This seems like a set up to protect the one who is making the prediction. By making such a statement, one can insist extreme measures are necessary because of how bad things will be. If it turns out not to be as bad as predicted, the one making the predictions can claim it was because of the "interventions" that were done, no matter how severe or mild. But until we know what the outcome is, others

can use these predictions to impose their power i.e. declare an emergency, force businesses to close, impose shelter in place, etc., and force others to do things that may not be necessary or tolerated without fear or an emergency order. Those who make predictions should be held accountable, and specifically state what intervention to which they are referring, how much each will decrease infections or deaths, and why or how each intervention will decrease infections, seriousness of infections or deaths. This way, they can be held accountable and the leaders who rely on their predictions, are better able to evaluate risks vs. benefits so they can make better policy decisions.

- Disclose the accuracy of past predictions made by the group making the current prediction. If none were ever made, disclosing that too. If predictors have made accurate predictions in the past, it seems reasonable that their current prediction may be more reliable. If all their previous predictions have been wrong, or off by a significant factor, it may be understandable not to put too much credence in their current prediction.

There is nothing wrong with making mistakes if they were unavoidable if, when the prediction is made, the one making the predictions clearly indicates the likelihood of the prediction being wrong and the magnitude of the error. To those who make predictions, this may seem too harsh, but it is important. Everyone should have a certain amount of accountability. When someone makes a prediction that can have enormous health and financial impact, they better be accurate or at least accountable for how close it is to accuracy. Perhaps they need to state the statistical significance or confidence interval of their findings. Perhaps indicate the "factor of error" that may exist i.e. the chances that the actual death count may be 10% more or less is 20%. Or state that there is a 95% chance that the margin of error will be wrong by 100% or more. Such statements would be useful to those who rely on such predictions to make decisions, or policies that may affect millions or billions of people. This is not always done but needs to be.

Let us look at some examples that illustrate how important likelihood and magnitude are. If a chest X-ray shows a spot on your lung and your doctor says that it is probably not cancer. That is good news but what does probably mean? Does that mean 1%, 10%, 50% chance? Should you not worry about it or should you start planning for surgery, chemotherapy, or end of life decision? I believe you would want to know more exact information and the limitations of the information if they are present. That makes sense. If the doctor says, this a concerning finding and we need to do a CT scan and a biopsy as it is highly suspicious. If there is 30-50% chance of cancer and if cancer, an 80% chance of dying within 5 years, one would rush to get a CT scan and biopsy. Yet, if the doctor said, we see this kind of "incidental" finding frequently and it is rarely ever a problem. If the doctor informs the patient that such a finding only needs a follow up X-ray in 3-6 months to make sure it is not changing, then it would be reasonable to wait 3-6 months and not rush to have a scan done. If the physician tells you there is less than a 1 in 10,000 chance that it is cancer and even if it ultimately turns out to be cancer or happens to get bigger on a follow up X-ray, it is 95-100% curable, you are much less likely to be worried and afraid, or panic. This demonstrates the importance of knowing the likelihood and magnitude.

Now let us use another medical example. Say you go to the doctor because you accidentally smashed the tip of your finger. The doctor takes an X-ray that does not show a fracture but tells you that he does not see a fracture (not think it is broken) but says that there is a 10-20% chance that there could still be a fracture that he does not see on the x-ray. He mentions a CT, MRI or bone scan may be better at showing if a fracture exists. But then adds, "even if it is broken, we would not treat it any differently. It will eventually heal and should not cause any problem." Even though the chance of a fracture still being present is not insignificant, it really is not concerning because the consequences, or the magnitude" of the consequences, are not significant. It will get better and treatment is the same i.e. time. What is the purpose of getting a scan, spending more money, etc. if it will not make any difference as to the treatment or outcome? FYI, if a fracture is not in joint and at the end of a digit (finger or toe) and not at risk for getting infected (skin is not broken or possibility of contamination) or other complicating factors, no significant management of the fracture is necessary.

Some Perspective

One of the worst pandemics on record for the United States was the "Spanish Flu" in 1918-1919. This was caused by the H1N1 virus thought to come from birds (avian origin). It is estimated to have infected 500 million people worldwide which is believed to be about 1/3 of the world population at that time. It is estimated to have killed 50 million people worldwide and 675,000 people in the United States. As is often the case with viruses, mortality was higher in the young (under 5 years old) and the elderly (65 and older).[lxxxv]

Now let us look at what the Imperial College of London had estimated mentioned earlier. Without interventions, they expected 7.0 billion people to be infected by COVID-19. For accuracy, one does not become infected from COVID-19, they become infected from SARS-CoV-2 or coronavirus. Were they suggesting that 7 billion people were not only going to become infected but were going to have the "illness" caused by SARS-

CoV-2? Is one to assume that "illness" includes anyone with an infection, whether they have symptoms or signs of an illness or not. As we clarified early on, COVID-19 is not the virus, it is the illness caused by the virus. It would seem ridiculous to label someone who has no signs of illness as suffering from an illness or disease. We do not label people as having "Rhinovirus Disease 2019" because they might test positive for one of the viruses, or have antibodies to the Rhinovirus, that causes a common cold.[lxxxvi] Having said that, according to worldometers.info, the current world population is approximately 7,794,000,000.[lxxxvii] The US Population is approximately 332,639,102,[lxxxviii]

Based on these figures, it appears that 1 out of every 10 people infected with the Spanish flu in 1918-1919 died from it (10% mortality rate for those infected known as the Infection Fatality Rate). If the type of lethality that occurred with the Spanish Flu occurred today with Coronavirus, based on Imperial College estimation of 7 billion possibly infected, we would expect 700,000,000 worldwide deaths. This is calculated using a 10% mortality rate for anyone infected that seemed to occur with the Spanish flu (50 million of the 500 million infected died-an Infection Fatality Rate of 10%).

Based on the Imperial College of London's predictions of 7.0 billion out of approximately 7.79 billion getting infected if no interventions, that implies about an 89.8% infection rate of the population. Applying that rate to the United States population, one would expect that about 298.7 million people would get infected in the United States if SARS-CoV-2 had the same infectivity in the US and worldwide. If SARS-CoV-2 is as "lethal" as the Spanish Flu, one would expect approximately 29.8 million deaths in the US alone from the virus.

Let me give a non-medical example that illustrates chances or odds. Think of horses in horse racing. Of the horses racing, there may be certain horses that are favored to win i.e. 2:1 or 5:4 odds for horse A or B. There may also be horses that are long shots to win with odds of 30:1 or 45:1 (Horse C & D). So, before the race starts, we can be somewhat confident that one of the two "favorites" will win and somewhat confident that horse C or D will not win. These "odds" help us make better informed decisions. Why not do the same with predictions of things with greater ramifications than money?

Using the approximate number of 125,000 COVID-19 deaths as of June 27, 2020, and the estimated population of the United States of 328,000,000 in 2019, the number of death that have already occurred thus far is about 1 person in 2,600 people. While no one should ignore SARS-CoV-2 and the illness and death that it can cause i.e. COVID-19, one must also understand the facts and data available to us.

Keep in mind, greater than 90% of all deaths caused by SARS-CoV-19 affect people 55 years of age and older. If we count 10% (closer to 8%) of the approximate total deaths as of June 27, 2020, and use 12,500 instead of 125,000, the number of deaths in people 54 years old and younger, the mortality rate is approximately 1 in 26,000 in 54-year-olds and younger. This is not exact as we would have to lessen the population used for the calculation to only include 54-year-olds and younger (not entire US population). Even so, the number would still be far less than the approximate 1 in 4,000 to 1 in 8,000 chance each year of being killed in a car accident[lxxxix] or the approximate 1 in 4,824 chance of dying from a drug overdose. This was calculated using an estimated population of 325,000,000 in 2018 and dividing by the CDC data of 67,367 drug overdose deaths in 2018.[xc]

While no one should think COVID-19 is something to ignore or not to be concerned about, it does not appear that SARS-CoV-2 has the same mortality rate of the Spanish Flu of 1918-1919.

The infection mortality rate is not even close. The question to ask is: was the magnitude of the response warranted? This is a complicated question with many factors involved and will be more thoroughly discussed in Part 2 of this book series: *Lockdown 2020: Consequences & Perspective*.

From observing what is shown and stated on television, it appears that the media does not do a great job of providing all the facts or emphasizing facts that would be useful and valuable to viewers. It seems that they want to promote how bad things are and how things are getting worse without giving perspective. They spend a disproportionate amount of time and coverage on something (SARS-CoV-2) that does not kill nearly as many people as other conditions and diseases i.e. heart disease, cancer. The media seems interested in getting the "shock" effect, perhaps as a means of getting higher ratings. A few examples:

- The media fails to discuss specifically how deaths are measured and how the criteria to categorize deaths from COVID-19 was changed that resulted in significantly higher numbers that gives the appearance of more deaths
- Media fails to properly explain how excess deaths are assumed to be from COVID-19 or how the numbers can be artificially inflated (or reduced)
- Media fails to clarify what terms mean. When the term "actual" cases, one might assume that this is the actual or real number of deaths. They do a poor job of clearly explaining that it is an estimate and not the real count or what many would consider "actual", based on assumptions that are likely inaccurate.
- Media seem to be confused, not understand, or try to confuse the public by using SARS-CoV-2, virus, cases, and Coronavirus interchangeably with COVID-19. They

often state that people "catch COVID-19" when in fact one "catches" the virus or SARS-CoV-2 and may or may not develop illness. Does illness include people with zero symptoms who would not know they carry the virus? While this may seem picky to some, it seems odd that those who are supposed to deliver the news or important information to the public are not more concerned about getting things correct and communicating clearly to the public. Some believe the media has an obligation to do this. But that is another story and not the purpose of this book. The media does a poor job of explaining that COVID-19 is not the virus, but the illness caused by the virus. When they talk about 40,000 or 50,000 new cases diagnosed each day, they then shift and talk about how serious COVID-19 is. Some even use the term COVID-19 when taking about the newly diagnosed cases. They are quite different. Only a fraction of "coronavirus cases" develop COVID-19 (illness). Many people infected with SARS-CoV-2 have no idea they are infected; they have no symptoms.

To illustrate this point, during an episode of CNBC's *Crisis in America* that was hosted by Scott Wapner that aired on June 18, 2020, the host spoke with Sandra Morgan, Chairwoman and Executive Director of the Nevada Gaming Control Board. He asked her something to the effect of whether she was concerned about the "alarming" rise in cases regarding the re-opening of the casinos in Nevada. During that episode, statistics were shown on the screen that are shown in Table #3.

Table 3

State	New Cases	7 Day Average	Testing	Opening Day
Nevada	Up 100.24%	Up 29.12%	Up 332.66%	May 9
California	Up 161.95%	Up 13.34%	Up 264.77%	May 8
Oklahoma	Up 195.13%	Up 106.13%	Up 484.55%	April 24
Florida	Up 129.29%	Up 78.32%	Up 252.95%	May 4

*Information that was shown on *Crisis in America*, which aired on CNBC on June 18, 2020

As one can see, there was indeed a rise in the number of cases diagnosed in Nevada since the opening on May 9, 2020, as the host implied and/or stated. These are cases of SARS-CoV-2, not COVID-19. I believe the host stated that the number of cases doubled, or that it increased 100%. What the host failed to mention was the magnitude of the increase in testing. As one can see, the number of cases for Nevada was up 100.24% for the period after opening day on May 9, but the number of testing had increased by 332.66%. All other things being equal, this is not necessarily bad news, but could be a good thing. You are testing 332% more people and the number of positives is only increasing by 100%, less than 1/3 of what one might expect, all other things being equal. If the same amount of people were infected and you test twice as many people, you expect the number to double. If you test 300% more people, one expects a 300% increase in the people who test positive. But the increase in cases was less than one-third the increase in tests performed.

Forget SARS-CoV-2 for a minute. Let us use an example involving blood types. Let us assume a stadium of 100,000 people and 10,000 of them have the blood type AB+ (a 10% prevalence). If you randomly tested 10,000 people, you would expect 1,000 positives for AB+. Now if you increased the number of tests by 332% and tested 43,200 people, you would expect 4,320 cases, which is 432% of the previous amount, or 332% more than 1,000. So, if we tested 332% more people in Nevada, if the infection remained constant, one would expect a 332% rise in cases, not a third of that. One could argue there was a "decline" in relative, or expected, cases by about 65-70%. I am not sure whether the host intentionally was trying to make things seem "alarming," does not understand statistics, was instructed to ignore common sense, did not pay attention or there was some other reason, but my point is he seemed to only emphasize how bad things were, and not look at things from a different perspective.

It is possible that testing may be on asymptomatic people, where earlier tests may have been with symptomatic or ill patients, or there could have been some other bias involved. This is possible but was not mentioned during the discussion. But it is possible this was not the case, or that all other factors were the same. I am bringing this up as it was not mentioned on the episode. My point is that no one bothered to explain or clarify. It appeared there was a bias to make a point that things were "alarming." I am not trying to criticize any one host or representative of the media, I just happened to see this episode and record the data.

It is certainly reasonable to protect the typically vulnerable young and elderly, and practice good hygiene of hand washing, isolating, or quarantining those at risk, and disinfecting thoroughly. The same measures that were done in 1918 and 1919 when they had no vaccine or pharmaceutical treatments.

Wearing masks (and respirators) and social distancing can be added to this list. Had we done this early on, many lives may have been saved. Now that we have learned more, we know that the young are not especially at risk and do not need extra precautions as the elderly do.

Final thought is predictions often change. Predictions are highly dependent on information. If you use bad information when making calculations, you often get bad (inaccurate) predictions. As we discussed earlier, it is understandable if the information is bad or incomplete, the predictions will likely be wrong. If this is the case, it is imperative that those who make the predictions clearly communicate this to the public and leaders who use the information to make decisions that will affect the masses. As information becomes more accurate and complete, the predictions should also become more accurate. This is nothing new to anyone familiar with statistics, epidemiology, sports handicapping, meteorology, actuarial work, or any other type of forecasting and predicting.

As more people are tested, if more people with milder cases, (asymptomatic), are identified, than it is likely the case fatality rate will fall (percentage of people diagnosed who die). Mortality rate of the nation will likely rise as more people die, especially if hospitals become full or overwhelmed. If this does not happen but is assumed in predictions, the predictions may overestimate true deaths. If younger people are diagnosed in comparison to older people, the case mortality rate (IFR) will likely fall since older patients are more likely to progress to COVID-19 and ultimately die. The more underlying conditions that those infected with SARS-CoV-2 have (i.e. hypertension, diabetes, cancer, etc.), the more likely those patients will develop COVID-19 or severe illness and are at risk of death. This is would likely cause the case mortality rate to rise.

Chapter Three:

Diagnostic Testing

During this pandemic, one often hears of the need for "testing." Particularly during the first few weeks, there were regular calls for testing, criticism of political leaders and governmental agencies. In general, having accurate testing is useful for diagnosing, treating, managing patients, better understanding an illness, tracking the spread or containment of an infection, making more accurate predictions, and giving the public a sense of security and comfort. The key word is "accurate." If a test in inaccurate, it can lead to poor decisions, inaccurate predictions, and a false sense of security. Keep in mind, few if any tests are 100% accurate and even if a test is not great, it does not mean that it has no value. As with most things, one must consider the benefits of the tests and the results that it provides versus the risks of getting inaccurate information.

So how many tests are there? According to the FDA's website as of June 27, 2020, there are over 110 tests authorized to be used under the Emergency Use Authorization. Because of the pandemic and the great demand and outcry for testing by politicians, those in the medical field and the public, and because there was not enough testing available to meet demand during the declared public emergency, the Food and Drug Administration (FDA) began to authorize use of tests that are not approved under what is known as an Emergency Use Authorization (EUA) authority. The EUA authority allows the FDA to help strengthen the nation's public health protections against chemical, biological, radiologic, and nuclear threats during public health emergencies.[xci]

> "Under section 564 of the Federal Food, Drug, and Cosmetic Act, the FDA Commissioner may allow unapproved medical products or unapproved uses of approved medical products to be used in an emergency to diagnose, treat, or prevent serious or life-threatening diseases or conditions caused by chemical, biological, radiologic, or nuclear threat agents when there are no adequate, approved, and available alternatives. Section 564 of the FD&C Act was amended by the Project Bioshield Act of 2004, further amended by the Pandemic and All-Hazards Preparedness Reauthorization Act of 2013, the 21st Century Cures Act of 2016, and Public Law 115-92 of 2017."[xcii]

When an EUA authority is used during a declared emergency, it is not "approved." It is "authorized" or allowed to be used. In emergencies, a lower level of evidence is required for a test to be allowed than what is normally required for a test to be approved. During a declared emergency, manufacturers only need to show that a test "may be effective" as opposed to the usual requirement to "demonstrate safety and effectiveness."[xciii] If the declared emergency ends, any test authorized under the EUA authority would have to meet the higher threshold of approval i.e. demonstrate safety and effectiveness. You may also be interested to learn that during the emergency, many of the manufacturers of the testing equipment submitted the minimum number of samples required (60) and mostly did not use real samples from people, Instead, they used mostly lab-produced specimens of the virus.[xciv] Some might argue that by doing so, many tests that are subpar or may not be very effective under real-life, imperfect, circumstances of real specimens from real patients. In the real world, these tests may yield results worse than the "controlled" specimens used to meet the reduced threshold to get the tests to be authorized.

While EUA has its share of potential drawbacks, the reasoning for allowing a lower threshold to allow the test to be used is that it speeds up the process. It allows for more availability of tests that may be needed but unavailable. Ordinarily, to get a test approved (as opposed to being allowed to be used) may take extra weeks, months, or years. Governmental bureaucracy and inefficiency often cause delays in approval. The EUA is a way to speed up the ordinary slow process during times of an emergency. Whether the outcome is always good can be debated. It depends on the circumstances, but the intention of the EUA seems to be good.

It was mentioned that over 110 tests were made available for SARS-CoV-2 screening and/or testing under the EUA between February 29, 2020 and June 26, 2020. A complete list of these tests, including name, type, and manufacturer along with the date is available on the FDA's website. I will mention only a few of them here chronologically.

February 4, 2020. The CDC was allowed under the EUA authority to use its CDC 2019-Novel Coronavirus (2019-nCoV) Real-time RT-PCR Diagnostic Panel test. This is a molecular test and the first allowed under the EUA for SARS-CoV-2.

February 29, 2020. This was the second test allowed under the EUA for SARS-CoV-2 and was also a molecular test of Wadsworth Center NYDOH, the New York SARS-CoV-2 Real Time Reverse Transcriptase (RT)-PCR Diagnostic.

March 16, 2020. The first home collection test was authorized for another molecular test made by Laboratory Corporation of America called the COVID-19 RT PCR Test.

April 1, 2020. The first serology test (antibody test) authorized under the EUA was authorized for Cellex Inc. for its qSARS-CoV-2 IgG/IgM Rapid Test.

April 15, 2020. The first ELISA antibody test was authorized for SARS-CoV-2 under the EUA to Mount Sinai Laboratory for its COVID-19 ELISA IgG Antibody Test.

May 8, 2020. The first Antigen test was authorized under the SARS-CoV-2 EUA to Quidel Corporation for its Sofia 2 SARS Antigen FIA.

June 2, 2020. The first immunoassay test for SARS-CoV-2 under the EUA was authorized to Roche Diagnostics for its Elecsys IL-6.

June 26, 2020. The most recent test authorized by the FDA under the EUA for SARS-CoV-2 was for Inform Diagnostics for its molecular test called Inform Diagnostics SARS-CoV-2 RT-PCR Assay.

As you can see, there are different types of test. Many laypersons may call the different type of tests, nasal or oral swabs, or blood tests. I will list the specific types and try to explain them without getting too technical. It can be confusing even to physicians. For those who are interested, I am including this discussion for completeness. A more accurate way to identify tests is by what they test and how they do it. There are molecular and serologic tests. Within these two main categories, there are different types as well.

Molecular Tests

Molecular tests are used to test for active infection. For Coronavirus, this is typically done with a swab.

PCR Test. The reverse-transcription polymerase chain reaction (rRT-PCR) test looks for genetic material of the SARS-CoV-2 virus. This is the most common type of test that screens for active infection by SARS-CoV-2. The "success" of these tests depends on experience and expertise of the laboratory personnel, laboratory environment and the type and condition of the specimen being tested.

Antigen Test. This test looks for proteins found on or within the coronavirus rather than genetic material of the virus itself. The test for Strep throat happens to be an antigen test, also collected by swab. This is a point of care test allowing for faster results.[xcv]

Isothermal Nucleic Acid Amplification. This test is different from the PCR test and the method used in the Abbott ID NOW point of care test. "Isothermal amplification of nucleic acids is a simple process that rapidly and efficiently accumulates nucleic acid sequences at constant temperature."[xcvi] It is an alternative to PCR testing and are used for biosensing targets such as DNA, RNA, cells, proteins, small molecules, and ions.

Serology Test

Serology tests are used to detect previous infection, even if the person was never symptomatic. These are typically blood tests. These tests should not be used as the sole basis to diagnose or exclude SARS-CoV-2 infections. They test for either the IgM or the IgG (or can be both) antibodies to the SARS-CoV-2 virus. IgM antibodies are typically one of the first antibodies that a person develops after being infected. IgG antibodies typically are produced by the body after IgM antibodies and remain detectable for months or years.[xcviii]

One type is called a "**lateral flow**" that change color on a paper strip if antibodies are present.

ELISA tests. According to the CDC, the Enzyme-linked immunosorbent assay (ELISA) test is a blood test that is used to detect the presence and concentration of specific antibodies to the SARS-CoV-2 virus.

Neutralizing Antibody Test. This type of test is used to measure antibodies that are capable of "neutralizing" the virus and can prevent future infections. In support of the National Expanded Access Program for Convalescent Plasma research efforts, the Mayo Clinic has launched a SARS-CoV-2 neutralizing antibody test to try to develop a vaccine and effective therapies against SARS-CoV-2.[xcix] How neutralizing antibodies (NAbs) are thought to work is by blocking spike glycoproteins. The surface of the SARS-CoV-2 is coated with spike glycoproteins that bind with receptors located on the surface of healthy human cells. This allows the virus to enter the healthy human cell and infect the human cell leading to infection of that cell and any other cell it enters throughout the body. NAbs are produced by human B cells after the SARS-CoV-2 infects a person. Once NAbs are produced, they attack the spike glycoprotein and block the spike glycoprotein's binding ability, thus preventing the coronavirus virus from entering other healthy cells, thus preventing further or future infection. At the time of this writing, it is unknown how much, or what level of, NAbs is necessary to confer protective immunity, or how long such immunity may last.[c]

It was reported that

> "A recent study showed that neutralizing from a convalescent SARS patient could block the SARS-CoV-2 from entering into target cells in vitro, which implies a potential cross-protective epitope between the two viruses (SARS-CoV-1 and SARS-CoV-2). Thus, the potential immune protection against reinfection with SARS-CoV-2 may share some common features with convalescent SARS-CoV (SARS-CoV-1)"[ci]

While this is no guarantee that it will work in people, it is encouraging. Of course, we still need to know what levels of NAbs are needed to be effective and how long these antibodies will last. From studies of the SARS-CoV-1, "IgG and neutralizing antibodies were highly correlated and peaked 4 months after the onset of disease and deceased gradually thereafter."[cii] The same source "suggested that the immune responses of specific antibodies were maintained in more than 90% of recovered SARS-CoV (SARS-CoV-1) patients for 2 years."[ciii] Given the similarities between the two SARS-CoV (1 & 2), this demonstrates the possibility that immunity may be possible with the SARS-CoV-2. Obviously, not enough time has passed to know if there will be antibodies to the SARS-CoV-2 for 2 years after infection as appears to be the case for SARS-CoV-1, or if they will provide immunity to the person.

We do not know the accuracy of many of these tests. Many tests used in medicine are not especially accurate. Some argue that the tests are often wrong and do not, or should not, necessarily change how patients are treated. They argue that physicians should use their clinical judgment and not rely on imperfect tests. Others say the combination of the two are better without giving too much weight to the test results. The test for Strep throat has a sensitivity of 86% and the CDC reports that the "rapid flu tests are even worse, with a sensitivity ranging from 50-70 percent."[civ] Sensitivity is a measure of how well a test is able to detect people who are infected (positive cases).[cv] As one can see, common tests, that we are accustom to hearing their names that some may perceive as being definitive, are not very good at identifying the illness they are intended to diagnose. As many as half of people who have the flu may test negative. The test for coronavirus may not be much better, or could be worse. "Months into the outbreak, no one really knows how well many of the screening tests work."[cvi] "For now, most COVID-19 tests in the U.S. do not give data on real world performance, including how often the tests falsely clear patients of infection or falsely detect the virus."[cvii] Anecdotally, I asked many fellow emergency physicians on a blog that over 30,000 physicians can access, what test they used and what the sensitivity of that specific test was, and few replied with an answer as to the type of test they were performing. Even less could provide what the sensitivity of the test was. Of the ones who did provide a sensitivity, most or all were not sure of the exact sensitivity. A test with a 90% sensitivity, which is very good by many test standards, is not high enough to rely upon with something that can be as serious as an infection that can easily spread and harm many vulnerable people. It is believed that many, and possibly all of the current allowed tests for SARS-CoV-2, have sensitivities much lower than 90%. A negative test may be wrong and would give a false sense of security.

Given the accuracy, or lack thereof depending on how you look at it, tests are not too useful for the purposes of determining treatment for an individual, particularly if you do not require hospitalization. Despite their non-ideal accuracy, they still have some value for determining prevalence of the virus and tracking purposes. The reason I say testing is not too useful clinically is because it probably will not, or should not, change how the patient is treated. As of July 1, 2020, I am not aware of any approved recommendation by the FDA or reputable medical body, or any convincing evidence, to prescribe a medication to treat people in an outpatient setting whether they test positive or negative for SARS-CoV-2, whether with or without symptoms. Here are some scenarios that may explain why testing individuals in the "clinical" setting makes little to no difference in treatment of, or instructions to, the patient:

- Asymptomatic patient and test positive. No treatment necessary. Person should isolate self to avoid spreading virus. Should practice distancing and wear a mask. Notify health professional if something changes.

- Asymptomatic patient and tests negative. No treatment necessary but still no guarantee that it was not a false negative. Person could still be an infected carrier, and spread the virus. So should still practice distancing and wear a mask when cannot properly distance. Notify health professional if something changes.
- Symptomatic patient but not require hospitalization and tests positive. No pharmacologic treatment recommended. Person should isolate self to avoid spreading virus. Should practice distancing and wear a mask. Follow up with health professional and notify them if something changes.
- Symptomatic patient but not require hospitalization and tests negative. No pharmacologic treatment recommended. Person should isolate self to avoid spreading illness or the virus. Should practice distancing and wear a mask. Follow up with health professional and notify them if something changes.
- Patients requiring hospitalization. This may justify testing on the patient.
  - If test positive. (we are assuming that it is not a false positive)
    - Dexamethasone may benefit patients, particularly those who are severely ill i.e. require supplemental oxygen or mechanical ventilation
    - Hydroxychloroquine may benefit hospitalized COVID-19 patients
  - If test negative. This is where it becomes tricky. If the patient shows symptoms of, and is suspected of having COVID-19, is it reasonable to withhold a medication or treatment that is believed to be beneficial to COVID-19 patients knowing that the test

we are using is far from perfect? i.e.
Hydroxychloroquine or dexamethasone

If we believe a treatment benefits a hospitalized COVID-19 patient (based on Dexamethasone and hydroxychloroquine studies), believe a patient has COVID-19 clinically, and know the test for SARS-CoV-2 which is the virus that causes COVID-19 is not good, is it ethical to withhold treating a patient with hydroxychloroquine if hospitalized, or dexamethasone if on mechanical ventilation or requiring supplemental oxygen? These are the questions that we must ask? For those who somehow feel better having a test result, even if unreliable, go ahead and get one. But should the result of an unreliable test determine what is done for a patient that could potentially die, and that could significantly benefit from the medication? Add to this a couple other points. The side effects of either medications were not shown to be significant in the studies. And, we are not sure if a positive test is necessarily accurate. These are some of the real-life challenges that treating physicians must face. No test is perfect and the worse a test is, the less value it has. We cannot let bad data lead us to making bad decisions.

If someone tests negative and assumes, they do not have it, they may not avoid being around others i.e. an older person, parent, or grandparent, and unintentionally spread the virus. If you are a healthcare worker, you could spread it to vulnerable patients in a hospital that could potentially lead to serious infections and death. So, the negative test is nice but how much does it really change what is done for patients or those who may be exposed to others, particularly the vulnerable. The safest thing to do is to assume everyone is positive and act accordingly i.e. take precautions.

One would expect that the test makers to endorse their products. For example, Abbott Laboratories has a test mentioned earlier called the rapid ID Now test. It provides results within about 15 minutes. This is allegedly the test that is used at the White House to screen President Trump, his staff, and visitors. Abbott alleges studies have shown their test to "successfully detect between 91% and 95% or more of the virus cases when compared to other tests."[cviii]

"A preliminary report by New York University found the Abbott ID NOW test missed between one third and one half of infections caught by a rival test in patients screened for the virus."[cix] If the rival test that it was compared to has a sensitivity of 80% that would imply the Abbott test may detect as few as 40% of patients who have the virus. (50-70% of 80%=40-56%). Researchers at Stanford University, Loyola University and the Cleveland Clinic reports have also flagged problems with Abbott's ID NOW's accuracy.[cx] In the same article, the Mayo Clinic's Dr. Colin West "worries doctors and patients have put too much confidence in the current crop of tests, when an unknown number of patients with COVID-19 are likely receiving false negative results."[cxi] An NBC article indicated that 10 medical centers were contacted and 7 out of 10 of them reported not using Abbott's test. "All seven cited issues with accuracy."[cxii] Accuracy is a big deal and very important, particularly when the consequences of a misdiagnosis can result in significant harm. "Even a modest error rate can have grave consequences during an outbreak like COVID-19. West (Dr. Colin West of the Mayo Clinic) gives the example of a test that is 95% accurate at detecting the virus and is used on a million people would result in 50,000 people being incorrectly"   diagnosed. Keep in mind, I am not aware of any SARS-CoV-2 screening tests currently being used that are anywhere near as good as 95%. Perhaps 80% is closer to what the better ones correctly diagnose, and some may be considerably lower 40-50%.

There are several reasons why the tests may not be as accurate as we would hope. The most likely ones most likely would be due to problems with the collection of the specimen, the timing of the collection of the specimen, the experience of the laboratory staff and the test itself.

Reasons for Poor Test Results:
Specimens Samples

Swabs are often used for nasopharyngeal and oropharyngeal samples. The SARS-CoV-2 preferentially infects and reproduces in the back of the nose (inner cavities). If you swab the wrong area, you could miss getting a specimen that has the SARS-CoV-2. In addition, it the virus does not happen to be there i.e. moved elsewhere in the body such as the lungs and no longer in the throat, the nasopharyngeal swab may come up negative even though the patient is infected. These tests are uncomfortable for the patient and therefore optimal samples may not be obtained. These tests are PCR tests. Another test that avoids this discomfort is a saliva test. Unfortunately, an oral specimen of saliva may miss up to 50% of asymptomatic positive patients.[cxiv]

Laboratory Personnel

If the personnel collecting the specimens do not test the correct location, do not get an adequate sample, or do not follow the recommended collection technique, it is more likely the result will be inaccurate. I.e. do not use correct swab, store in wrong container, etc.

Timing

According to Dr. Lauren Kucirka, a medical resident at Johns Hopkins and lead author of a study published in Annals of

<u>Internal Medicine,</u> testing too early after exposure to the virus substantially raises the risk of a false negative result.[cxv] According to Dr. Kucirka's study, testing three days after the onset of symptoms is when the test is most likely to be valid.[cxvi] It is unclear which specific test that was used in that particular study and if this timing would apply to other tests? A big drawback of such guidance is with asymptomatic patients. Physicians will be unable to properly time the test in such patients, who are likely the largest group of people infected with SARS-CoV-2. I.e. infected but asymptomatic public.

Test Itself

Many tests that go through the regular approval process during non-declared emergencies (non EUA) are not great in their accuracy as already discussed i.e. Strep test, Influenza test. So, it is not difficult to believe that tests that undergo a less stringent process during an emergency may not "meet the same muster" or be as good as those that do. While some tests that are authorized under the EUA may be good, they do not have to meet the same threshold as those that get approved during normal times. One example is that the samples created in the lab for the EUA testing may be "better" specimens with higher concentrations of virus that are easier to detect. It is possible that if a normal, real life specimen were used that the test may not be good enough to detect the lower concentration of virus and may not have passed the lower authorization threshold. It is possible they would not meet the normal criteria that is required in the normal approval process.

I hope this testing section helps you understand the different tests, how they work and their limitations. Perhaps it may have even been interesting to some. If you do not understand everything about all the tests or cannot explain everything about them to someone else, do not get frustrated. Many within healthcare with years of experience may not know, or may have forgotten, many of the details. The good news is that there are tests available and we do not have to know everything about them. Of course, it is nice to know their accuracy and indications to help us understand the significance of the results that they give.

Testing Take Home Points

As mentioned, testing can be complicated. The take home message is there are a lot of different tests available, that check for the SARS-CoV-2 virus and things associated with a current or previous infection, that can be performed to help detect it or assist in making a diagnosis. No test available today is perfect. In fact, some may be rather poor at making an accurate diagnosis and in many cases, we are not sure what the accuracy (sensitivity or specificity) of many of these tests is. It is likely that more tests will be developed, some of the existing tests will go away, particularly if the normal approval criteria must be met i.e. if the declared emergency ends, and hopefully the accuracy will improve and approach 100%. Only time will tell.

Because of accuracy issues, testing has limited value on screening individual patients. Whether the test that may be flawed with accuracy issues is positive or negative will likely have little influence on treatment. Unless a person is clinically ill i.e. severe symptoms, short of breath, unable to eat, high fevers, etc., there is no specific "pharmacologic treatment" or interventions are indicated at this time. Patients that are not ill are given instructions such as eating healthy, staying well hydrated, rest, etc., to follow up and to notify physician if they get worse. If someone tests positive, they should avoid others and take precautions not to spread. But even if one is negative, they should still take precautions as if they are infected because many who are infected have no symptoms. That is why testing patients who are well has little effect on treatment or instructions and is not too helpful in well-appearing non-hospitalized people.

While the current tests are inaccurate and not great for screening of healthy or asymptomatic individuals, they are not without any value. Even screening tests that are not great can still help with collecting data that may help us understand how prevalent that virus is, how quickly it is spreading or how well it is being controlled. While not perfect, the data can give us an idea of trends and help us make some public health decisions (for the masses, not necessarily for the individual).

Testing, even if not as accurate as we would like may be helpful for individual patients who are ill, particularly the ones severely ill. The reason for this is dexamethasone, a steroid, my improve outcomes in patients who require supplemental oxygen or mechanical ventilation and hydroxychloroquine may improve survival in hospitalized patients. Thus, a positive test may change the treatment in this group of people (individuals who are ill or severely ill). Although, if a patient is severely ill and the test comes back negative, doctors may still decide to treat the patient in case the test results were wrong given their accuracy issues. The doctors may make the diagnosis based on signs, symptoms, and the current pandemic. In such a case, the doctor would be making a clinical diagnosis versus relying on a lab test or making a "lab test diagnosis".

Assume the worst but hope for the best. Assume almost everyone has the virus, so protect yourself and protect them. I say almost everyone because if I did not, someone would argue if everyone has it, there is no need for precautions because everyone already is infected.

- Practice good hygiene, wash your hands regularly and always before eating, touching your face, eyes, nose, mouth.
- Have hand sanitizer with you when you cannot wash your hands. I.e. after pumping gas, pushing a shopping cart, going to post office, etc.
- Use disinfectants and wipe surfaces, doorknobs, and everything else that anyone may touch. SARS-CoV-2 may survive for days on certain surfaces.
- Do not share drinking glasses, drinks, eating utensils or cigarettes. No one should smoke at all as smoking contributes to more deaths, by far, than SARS-CoV-2 or COVID-19 has caused, and has done so each year for decades.
- Social distancing with anyone you cannot be reasonably sure is not infected i.e. non-household persons.
- Wear a face mask or respirator. N95, surgical or cloth mask when around others, especially if indoors and cannot maintain safe distances (6 feet or more).
- Avoid sick contacts and if you are sick, stay home and isolate yourself from others.
- If you need to cough or sneeze, cover your mouth (even if wearing a mask) and then wash your hands afterwards.
- Use common sense and good judgment and be respectful of others.

We are all in this together. If we all do the right things, the chances we will get through this with less infections, illnesses, death, and suffering will be better.

Chapter Four:

COVID-19 Death Statistic

The first case of SARS-CoV-2 in the United States was confirmed on January 20, 2020. According to Johns Hopkins University, the number of confirmed cased of SARS-CoV-2 was 2,510,151 and the number of deaths in the United States from SARS-CoV-2 was 125,484 as of June 28, 2020. [cxvii]

The CDC reported similar numbers on the same date: 2,504,175 total cases and 125,484 total deaths. [cxviii]

In the first 6 months of the year and about 5 months since the first case was diagnosed in the US, over 125,000 people have "died" from COVID-19. In the last day (June 27, 2020), 44,703 new cases were diagnosed, and 508 deaths were attributed to COVID-19. [cxix]

The count is likely to increase further as more contract SARS-CoV-2 and COVID-19 every day and many others are currently hospitalized. Most of these patients will recovery, but some will unfortunately die.

SARS-CoV-2 and the disease that it causes, COVID-19, seem to affect those who are older. To get a better idea of how much it does, data was taken from the CDC's website, listed according to age groups, and is provided in the following charts. Table 4 and Table 5 have the same categories but represent two different time periods. Just to provide you with a couple snapshots in time, Table 4 is for the week ending June 24, 2020 and Table 5 is for the week ending May 13, 2020. The data applies for the entire United States.

Table 4

SARS-CoV-2 Statistics for the Week ending June 24, 2020[cxx]

Age of Person Being Counted	Number of COVID-19 Deaths	Number of All Deaths	Percentage of All COVID-19 Deaths	Number of Influenza Deaths
Under 1 year	9	6,504	0.008%	14
1-4 Years	6	1,259	0.006%	40
5-14 Years	13	1,859	0.012%	46
15-24 Years	132	11,608	0.122%	51
25-34 Years	732	24,675	0.678%	146
35-44 Years	1,860	35,202	1.72%	232
45-54 Years	5,238	66,547	4.85%	560
55-64 Years	12,895	155,823	11.94%	1,197
65-74 Years	22,429	239,025	20.77%	1,401
75-84 Years	28,735	296,558	26.61%	1,423
85 Years & Older	35,948	376,456	33.29%	1,334
All Ages	107,997	1,215,516	100%	6,444

*Figures may not be exact or reconcile due to rounding error

Table 5

SARS-CoV-2 Statistics for the Week ending May 13, 2020[cxxi]

Age of Person Being Counted	Number of COVID-19 Deaths	Number of All Deaths	Percentage of All COVID-19 Deaths	Number of Influenza Deaths
Under 1 year	4	4,258	0.007%	11
1-4 Years	2	832	0.004%	35
5-14 Years	6	1,223	0.011%	43
15-24 Years	59	7,452	0.107%	42
25-34 Years	388	15,975	0.707%	135
35-44 Years	973	22,887	1.77%	214
45-54 Years	2,772	44,291	5.05%	529
55-64 Years	6,725	106,004	12.26%	1,136
65-74 Years	11,524	164,217	21.01%	1,334
75-84 Years	14,930	206,121	27.21%	1,357
85 Years & Older	17,478	262,347	31.86%	1,274
All Ages	54,861	835,607	100%	6,110

*Figures may not be exact or reconcile due to rounding error

As you can see from Tables 4 & 5:

- Over 90% of all COVID-19 deaths occur in people 55 years of age and older i.e. 92.61% in the week ending June 24, 2020 and 92.34% in the week ending May 13, 2020.
- The number of deaths associated with Influenza seems low compared to the typical annual deaths attributed to

Influenza. The CDC indicates that Influenza typically is responsible for 12,000-61,000 deaths each year.[cxxii]

- It is possible some of the deaths attributed to COVID-19 may be due to Influenza
- Ages 75-84 had the highest percentage of deaths from COVID-19/SARS-CoV-2 compared to all deaths in their group compared to other age groups. It was 7.24% (14,930 out of 206,121 total deaths) in the week ending May 13, 2020, and 9.69% (28,735 out of a total of 296,558 deaths) in the week ending June 24, 2020.

It is not too surprising that many of the deaths are in the elderly populations. That is the case with the regular flu (Influenza A & B) and was the case with the Spanish Flu in 1918-1919. Viruses and other infections often seem to be "more dangerous" or cause more harm to the vulnerable i.e. those with underlying diseases, immunocompromised, and the age extremes, both young and old. One of the most unexpected things about SARS-CoV-2 is the young are not more affected (deaths) by the COVID-19. The number of deaths in those under 5 years of age made up about 1/100th of 1 percent of all COVID-19 deaths.

COVID-19 obviously causes a disproportionate amount of harm to the elderly. Tables 4 and 5 shows that over 90% of all COVID-19 related deaths were in people 55 years of age and older, 92.61% and 92.34% respectively. So, it should not be surprising that lots of death occurred in long term facilities i.e. nursing homes, adult care residences, and skilled nursing facilities. A high percentage of all COVID-19 deaths occurred in long term facilities. Many of these facilities have patients who are both elderly and have underlying medical conditions. According to an article published in May 2020, the following states had the following percentage of all COVID deaths in their respective state, occur in long term facilities:[cxxiii]

- New York, 20% of all deaths in state occurred in long term facilities. The highest absolute number of deaths of any state.
- New Jersey, 53% of all deaths in state occurred in long term facilities. The second highest absolute number of deaths of any state.
- New Hampshire, 72% of all deaths in state occurred in long term facilities
- Pennsylvania, 70% of all deaths in state occurred in long term facilities

To get a better perspective, it is useful to look at deaths from other causes i.e. Table 6. Doing so may give you a better perspective of how COVID-19 compares to other illnesses, diseases, and injuries. There are many other illnesses or conditions that kill people, and have been doing so for years, but do not seem to be getting as much attention from politicians, people in the media or in the headlines. To many, COVID-19 is scary. Perhaps it is because we do not have enough information about it i.e. fear of the unknown, or because we do not have enough perspective. It is my hope that this book and the following chart will help you get some perspective, so COVID-19 does not scare you. This is not to say we should ignore COVID-19, not take precautions, or not make good decisions. You should always do this. It is hoped that it will remove some of the fear and panic that many seem to have and allow people to be more at ease while still protecting themselves and others, be less emotional, use better judgment, and live happier, less stressful, healthy lives.

Table 6

Leading causes of death in 2017 from CDC[cxxiv] & HCHS[cxxv]

Cause of Death	Number of Deaths in 2017	*Mortality Rate for US Population ^(# deaths per 100,000 population)
Heart Disease	647,457	*1 in 502 people ^(199.2 deaths /100K)
Cancer	599,108	*1 in 543 people ^(184.3 deaths/100K)
Accidents (unintentional injuries)	169,936	*1 in 1913 people ^(52.3 deaths/100K)
Chronic Lower Respiratory Disease	160,201	*1 in 2029 ^(49.3 deaths/100K)
Cerebrovascular Accident (Stroke)	146,383	*1 in 2221 ^(45.0 deaths/100K)
Alzheimer's Disease	121,404	*1 in 2678 ^(37.3 deaths/100K)
Diabetes	83,564	*1 in 3890 ^(25.7 deaths/100K)
Influenza and Pneumonia	55,672	*1 in 5839 ^(17.1 deaths/100K)
Nephritis, Nephrotic Syndrome & Nephrosis	50,633	*1 in 6420 ^(15.6 deaths/100K)

Intentional Self-Harm (Suicide)	41,173	*1 in 7896 ^(12.7 deaths/100K)

*2017 United States Population of 325,084,758[cxxvi] was used for Mortality Rate calculation (number of people that includes 1 person who will die on average within that number)

^The number of deaths per 100,000 population is calculated using the formula:

Number of deaths from specific Cause/US population X 100,000 = (# deaths per 100,000 population)

- In 2017, a total of 2,813,503 resident deaths from all causes yielded a death rate of 863.8 per 100,000 population[cxxvii]
- 92.6 deaths/100,000 population for COVID-19 after adjusting for the complete year (using a 25,097 monthly death average, achieved by 125,484 COVID-19 deaths/5 month). The number of deaths per 100,000 population (after adjusting for shorter time-period) using 2017 population for COVID-19 is 92.6 deaths per 100,000 population. This assumes COVID-19 maintains same monthly average deaths that it did between January 21, 2020 and June 28, 2020.
- COVID-19 would rank third in expected deaths per 100,000 population between #4 Accidental injuries (52.3 deaths/100K population) and #2 Cancer (184.3 deaths/100K population)

As of this writing, 125,484 deaths have been assigned to COVID-19 / SARS-CoV-2 and would rank #6 on the annual death count for 2017. Granted, COVID-19 deaths have occurred in about a 6-month time frame. If we break down the number of deaths into a monthly average, heart disease would still be #1 at 53,954, Cancer #2 at 49,926 and COVID-19 at 25,097. There seems to be almost non-stop reporting about SARS-CoV-2 or COVID-19. Many are outraged more is not being done i.e. testing, treatments, vaccines. Many use the "deadliness" of COVID to justify shelter in place, forcing businesses to close or to justify the lockdown. Whether you believe this was indicated or not, the question is if we react to something that is causing about

25,000 deaths per month, why are not the same people reacting 4 times as much for heart disease and cancer? Each of these diseases kills about 2 times more per month than COVID-19 and have done so for years. Should we be having 4 times the news coverage for heart disease and cancer as we are having for COVID-19? Add to this, other non-COVID-19 causes of death likely cause more lost years of expected life than COVID-19. Should we be spending 4 times as much on heart disease and cancer as we are on COVID-19? Not suggesting we should or should not. Just giving you something to think about and to give some perspective. Does it matter what people die from? The result is the same, there is loss of life and many loved ones behind grieving.

Keep in mind, 25,000 deaths per month for COVID-19 may be a high estimation. Any death that is coded under the International Classification of Diseases (ICD) as ICD code UO7.1 on the death certificate, plus excess deaths are included in this number. If we only count confirmed cases, as many of the heart disease and cancer deaths are, the number of COVID-19 could potentially be cut in half. In case you are wondering, the ICD Code U07.1 stands for probable or presumed COVID-19, with or without lab confirmation. It is possible that some or many of the deaths attributed to COVID-19 may be incorrect and not ever "confirmed."

There have been anecdotal reports of deaths being attributed to COVID-19 if they test positive for SARS-CoV-2, regardless of the cause of death. Fr example, someone who has a heart attack and dies but tested positive for SARS-CoV-2, someone who died in a bad car accident that tested positive for SARS-CoV-2, or someone who sustained a gunshot wound and died who tested for SARS-CoV-2. It is believed that most would not consider these COVID-19 related deaths and should not be counted as such. I am not aware of any hard evidence that this is being done but mentioning for those who may be wondering.

One might worry that COVID-19 could increase even more. While this is possible and one should always consider it, the data from the CDC demonstrates that deaths peaked in mid-April and have consistently fallen each week since to the most recent week reported that ended June 20, 2020, which had 481 deaths. There are recent reports that the number of cases being diagnosed is increasing and could cause an increase in deaths. There is usually a delay between cases diagnosed and actual recovery or death, so the data may lag. Table 7 shows a weekly breakdown of COVID-19 deaths, all deaths, excess deaths (any amount higher than expected deaths) and influenza related deaths since tracking began with the week ending February 1, 2020. Keep in mind, according to NPR, the first case identified in the United States was confirmed by the CDC on January 20, 2020.[cxxviii]

Table 7

Analysis of COVID-19 & other Deaths from week ending February 1, 2020-June 20, 2020.[cxxix]

Week Ending Date in which Death Occurred	*All Deaths involving COVID-19	Death from All Cases	^Percent of Expected Deaths	~All Deaths Involving Influenza
2/1/2020	1	58,179	98	477
2/8/2020	1	58,771	98	516
2/15/2020	0	57,904	98	549
2/22/2020	5	57,864	100	557
2/29/2020	5	58,250	101	638
3/7/2020	33	58,515	101	620

3/14/2020	52	57,428	101	611
3/21/2020	551	58,059	102	543
3/28/2020	3,052	62,067	111	439
4/4/2020	9,504	70,838	127	461
4/11/2020	15,698	77,492	140	468
4/18/2020	16,350	74,839	138	260
4/25/2020	14,103	70,998	132	143
5/2/2020	11,670	65,877	123	62
5/9/2020	10,747	63,528	121	46
5/16/2020	8,772	59,998	115	19
5/23/2020	6,666	56,162	108	20
5/30/2020	5,445	52,943	101	10
6/6/2020	3,904	49,147	92	10
6/13/2020	2,148	40,134	73	7
6/20/2020	481	23,276	37	3
Total Deaths	109,188	1,232,269	106	6,459

*Deaths with confirmed or presumed COVID-19, coded to ICD-10 code U07.1. There can be a lag of 1-8 weeks or more from time of death and completion of death certificate depending on jurisdiction and cause of death.

^Percent of expected deaths is the number of deaths for all causes in the week in 2020 compared to the average number across the same week in 2017-2019. Analysis of 2015-2016 data found completeness is at least 75% complete within 8 weeks of when the death occurs. Anything above 100% expected deaths would be considered "Excess Deaths"

~Counts of deaths involving influenza include deaths with pneumonia or COVID-19 also as a cause of death.

One needs to clearly define what should be counted towards COVID-19 deaths. It seems straight forward that if someone contracts COVID-19 and dies primarily from complications of COVID-19, then that is a COVID-19 or COVID-19 related death. But what if someone during the COVID-19 pandemic stays at home because his employer was mandated to close i.e.

Governor or Mayor's order to close businesses deemed "non-essential" because of SARS-CoV-2, suffers from depression because of the isolation and commits suicide. Is this death attributed to depression? Or is it attributed to COVID-19? Some may say depression, others may argue COVID-19, yet others may argue it was the result of the politician's "policy" that mandated the shutdown. But such questions need to be clearly answered, categorized, and defined, if we wish to avoid confusion, or misleading the public. If someone dies in a car crash but was diagnosed with SARS-CoV-2, or even COVID-19 the day before, was the cause of death multi-trauma and hemorrhage or was it COVID-19, or both? Again, how one answers this question and others will determine whether you agree with how the CDC measures deaths from, related to, or caused by COVID-19.

A good example of this is prostate cancer in men. It is reported that the prevalence of prostate cancer in men over 60 years of age is about 50%.[cxxx] It may be higher. If we assume that half of men over 60 have prostate cancer, should we use prostate cancer as the cause of death in every one of them? Should prostate cancer be listed as the cause of 50% of all men 60 years old and older? A reasonable answer is no. It is my understanding that the CDC and others do not consider prostate cancer as the cause of death in every man who dies with prostate cancer (about 50% of the male population over 60). The same standard should apply to SARS-CoV-2. As with patients who have prostate cancer, patients who test positive or suspected of having SARS-CoV-2 can die with SARS-CoV-2 and not from SARS-CoV-2 or COVID-19. This may sound like a minor thing but can be substantial and distort reality.

But it is not completely clear exactly who is counted and if the numbers reflect the "real" numbers. One would think that when someone dies, the treating physician or coroner determines the "cause of death" and if the cause of death is listed as COVID-19, these numbers reflect the total number who meet these criteria. But I am not sure that is the case. Also, it is not clear if the "official" COVID-19 death count is deaths only caused by COVID-19 or COVID-19 was the main or primary cause of death. What if the patient happened to test for SARS-CoV-2 but had no COVID-19 symptoms? Is death assumed to be from COVID-19 for any reason i.e. no known reason, so "logic" says it must be from COVID-19? Knowing the answers to these and other questions will allow us to better determine if we believe the COVID-19 death toll accurately reflects the deaths caused by SARS-CoV-2 i.e. COVID related.

It is my understanding that the numbers listed on the CDC site are "provisional deaths." It is my understanding that this number is generated from data off of death certificates that are sent to the National Center for Health Statistics (NCHS) on a daily basis from all 50 states, Puerto Rico and the District of Columbia.[cxxxi] Keep in mind, provisional counts are subject to change. According the CDC:

- "Provisional data are not yet complete. Counts will not include all deaths that occurred during a given time period, especially for more recent periods. However, the completeness of the data can be estimated by examining the average number of deaths reported in previous years.
- Provisional counts are not final and are subject to change. Counts from previous weeks are continually revised as more records are received and processed.
- Death Counts should not be compared across states. Some states report daily deaths to NCHS, while other states report deaths weekly or monthly.

> State vital record reporting may also be affected or delayed by COVID-19 response activities."[cxxxii]

In fairness, sometimes it is hard to accurately measure things in real time, particularly when there is a pandemic and people are not properly prepared or have a set of rules that everyone follows. There is a risk of under reporting and over reporting. Perhaps as an attempt to compensate for what one may assume to be an undercount, those in charge create formulas or come up with new ways of counting the cause of deaths. It is hard to say. Here are some thoughts how the "official" death counts may be under, or over, counted. You decide if you think the way the death count is measured accurately reflects the number of deaths caused by COVID-19.

Possible factors that may cause the "real" number of deaths from COVID-19 to be under counted. As you notice, I intentionally did not use the term official number of deaths as we really do not know if the "official" count is higher than the true number of deaths caused by COVID-19, or whether it is lower than the true number of deaths caused by COVID-19. Assuming the death was "truly caused" by COVID i.e. the main reason for the death, here is a partial list of the reasons why the death may have been assigned a different cause of death, and cause the "official number" to be lower than the real, or true, number of deaths caused by COVID-19:

- Elderly who died may have be assigned a "natural" cause of death. i.e. in hospital, nursing home or at home i.e. it was not realized that they had cough, fever, shortness of breath, pneumonia, or respiratory distress and exposed to SARS-CoV-2, or others who had COVID-19. Not tested for SARS-CoV-2 but had symptoms of COVID-19.

- People may have been assigned a "different code" on their death certificate by the treating physician or coroner.
- Chronically ill person who died may have been assigned a cause of death from their underlying condition instead of COVID-19
- People had symptoms but assumed it was the flu and not COVID-19
- People may have died and be unaccounted for and thus never counted.
- People may have died and even though they were tested, the test falsely resulted as negative

Now let us assume the death was NOT from COVID-19 and consider possible reasons why the death was incorrectly counted as a COVID-19 related death. Put another way, a partial list why the official reported number of deaths may be higher than the "true" number of deaths caused by COVID-19:

- People who died from other causes were assumed to have COVID-19. I.e. if a patient had Influenza (regular "flu") and died, it may have been assumed to be COVID-19.
- If patient had multiple medical problems when died but happened to test positive for SARS-CoV-2, the cause of death may have been counted as COVID-19.
- If patient tested negative but the doctor assumed it was a false negative result, COVID-19 may have been listed as the cause of death when in fact it was a true negative test and the death was from some other cause.
- If a patient had symptoms of the flu, which could also have been from COVID, but no lab test confirmation, and assumed to be from COVID-19
  - This could be not testing for either the flu or COVID-19

- Testing only for the flu and it was negative, so it was assumed to be SARS-CoV-2 (even though it is reported that the flu test can be wrong 30-50% of the time)
- Testing only for COVID-19, results negative but still assume COVID-19
- Tested negative for the flu and SARS-CoV-2 but assumed to be SARS-CoV-2 since there is a SARS-CoV-2 (COVID-19) pandemic
- Provisional deaths are not strictly based on true deaths and death certificates but are "adjusted" and weighted to account for incomplete data.

- Excess deaths are assigned as COVID-19 related, even though could be from many other causes.

Excess death counts are defined by the CDC as "the difference between the observed numbers of deaths in specific time periods and expected number of deaths in the same time periods."[cxxxiii] These are often weekly averages that are then compared to weekly averages for the previous years. So, if the estimated number of deaths in one week in one jurisdiction i.e. city or state, etc., is 1,000 but the actual reported deaths is 1,500, that would count as 500 excess deaths. Using the excess deaths, these 500 extra deaths would be counted as due to COVID-19 and would be added to the excess death total from other jurisdictions. But if the actual number of deaths is 800, which would give a difference of -200, -200 would not be added (200 would not be deducted from the total of the other jurisdictions). Instead zero would be used.[cxxxiv] No negative numbers are used. This seems biased toward only elevating the number of COVID-19 deaths. What if COVID-19 caused people to leave town and move to an area that was not a hotspot, and ultimately died in the new city from something other than COVID-19 that may have been specific to the new city. Assume it was 500 people who moved from old city to the new city that died. These 500 deaths would likely be counted as deaths (COVID-19 related) in the new city since there would likely be "excess deaths" in that city (500 deaths of people that ordinarily would not occur). If the city they moved away from had fewer deaths than expected (500), that city would not be able to deduct that number from the excess that the new city contributed to the "excess death" total. The old city may have 500 fewer deaths than expected. Instead of reporting -500 deaths to the national total, it would have to be counted as zero, as negative numbers are not counted. It would seem reasonable that negative numbers should be allowed as the 500 additional deaths in the new city would be offset by the 500 lower deaths in the old city. Given the way negative numbers are not allowed, this could result in 500 deaths being "miscounted."

Another example of how the reported deaths may misrepresent actual causes is that it assumes the excess deaths are from COVID-19. If the actual number of weekly deaths are higher than the average number of weekly deaths over the past ten years, why do we assume it is from COVID-19? There is a saying about assuming. When you ASSuME, you make an "ass out of you and me." Having said that, I understand that is possible that some of the excess deaths are from COVID-19 during a pandemic, but to assume all are from COVID-19 is not a fact. There are causes other than infection by SARS-CoV-2 and COVID-19 that people can die from during a pandemic. So, how do we count the following?

- The difference of deaths from other causes related to the lockdown to try and "protect" us from the SARS-CoV-2 and developing COVID-19 itself?
- The people who die from substance abuse or overdoses?

- The people who commit suicide?
- Those who die because they did not seek out care out of fear of contracting COVID-19?
- People with chest pain that are having a heart attack stay at home out of fear that they may get COVID-19 and die when they might have lived had they went to the ER? Do we count these deaths from myocardial infarctions (heart attacks) or due to COVID-19?
- Victims of domestic abuse (spousal, child and other) who may perish because they were trapped in the same dwelling as their abuser.

This is not to say that all excess deaths are not from COVID-19, but it does not seem correct to assume all excess deaths are from COVID-19. To its credit, the CDC acknowledges on their website that the estimates of excess deaths "may not be due to COVID-19, either directly or indirectly.[cxxxv] Yet, these deaths are included in the figures for COVID-19 deaths. Why have a bias that seems to only be able to overestimate the number of deaths? Why not bias it in a way that minimizes the number? Why not count only a percentage of the excess deaths towards the "cause" that is getting the attention (currently SARS-CoV-2 or COVID-19)? The method being used seems to be biased towards the "virus" that is causing the fear and panic amongst the public. Unless one digs into the matter and researches, this information is not commonly known or mentioned consistently, if at all, on television when the death toll is reported. This is important information to know as the excess numbers can be significant.

Keep in mind, excess deaths are in addition to all COVID-19 deaths that are already counted. So this "count" is assigning cause of death based on assumptions and not on hard evidence, the examining physician's professional opinion or autopsy. It is based on assumptions and a formula. The validity of the assumptions can be questioned. Not exactly what some would call scientific or objective.

Another concern is there may be different criteria of how deaths from COVID-19 are measured by different people in different cities and states. Unless it is uniform or clearly explained, the data can be misleading and less useful. While it may be with good intention, some may intentionally manipulate the numbers or change the way that the "numbers are determined" to meet a goal or agenda. In a BBC article, it is reported that New York changed the way it was going to count COVID-19 deaths. It cites Governor Andrew Cuomo as stating "the CDC had changed guidelines for how coronavirus deaths were to be recorded." [cxxxvi] In the April 15, 2020 article, it stated that "New York City's death count has spiked to more than 10,000 after it reported 3,778 people who likely had COVID-19 but died without being tested." [cxxxvii] The article adds "The new figures, from the city's Health Department, mark a 60% rise in deaths." [cxxxviii] While it is possible that these extra deaths were from COVID-19, making a change in criteria that causes a 60% change in the figures seems quite significant. In a May 14, 2020 article, it is stated that "as of May 1, 2020 New York City reported 13,156 confirmed deaths and 5,126 probable deaths (deaths with COVID-19 on death certificates but no laboratory test performed) for a total of 18,282 deaths." [cxxxix] Another 5,148 additional excess deaths were added by the CDC. Thus, the total number of "Actual COVID-19 deaths as of May 1, 2020 in New York City" was reported as 23,430, even though there were only 13,156 confirmed cases. [cxl] Depending on how one views what constitutes COVID-19 being a "legitimate" cause of death, the statistics vary widely. The 23,430 number of "actual cases" calculated by the CDC is considerably more than 13,156 confirmed cases reported by New York City. It is 10,274 more deaths to be exact, or approximately 78% more than the number of confirmed deaths. Even if we count "probable deaths" which may or may not be from COVID-19, the CDC number is 5148 higher than the combined amount of confirmed and probable COVID-19 deaths, or over 28% higher than this number (18,282), which some may consider already inflated.

One must wonder if someone was changing the criteria to intentionally raise the numbers to meet some expected or pre-determined death toll. I am not trying to lessen the significance of death from any cause or trying to make an argument that SARS-CoV-2 should not be a concern. I am simply trying to bring this change in determining the cause of death, and the way deaths are counted to everyone's attention. This can be a serious matter as it may dramatically change the numbers and the perception of the significance of an illness or disease and have big financial, policy and political implications. Everyone needs to be aware of this because if you are not, you may think that there was an "explosion" of cases or a sudden worsening in the contagiousness or mortality of this virus and not simply due to an "accounting" or "definition" change. I.e. change in the manner counts are made likely resulted in significant total counts throughout the country. Changing the rules of accounting during a project will likely be confusing and possibly harmful. Recall the criteria was changed to "probable or presumed COVID-19, with or without lab confirmation" from requiring more "objective" criteria i.e. clinical evidence of COVID-19 and a positive test. By changing the criteria, it would be more likely to reach inflated prediction numbers that were done when the criteria was more stringent.

As a physician, sometimes it can be difficult to determine an accurate cause of death without an autopsy. Sometimes it is obvious, other times not so much. Let us start with a relatively simple example. If someone suffers a gunshot wound to the chest. The cause of death may be listed as catastrophic injury to the heart and major blood vessels, bleeding, low oxygen level from a hemothorax (blood in the thoracic cavity), etc. It would be hard to argue that the cause of death was from COVID-19, even if the victim had a positive SARS-CoV-2 test. But it is possible that someone could list it as a cause of death. Now a difficult one. If someone with very severe congestive heart failure (CHF) that requires a heart transplant gets pneumonia and had a heart attack. Any of the three could have killed this person. Was it the CHF that finally caused death or was it that he had a sudden heart attack that he could not handle? Was it the infection that caused it?

There is a saying that someone in college told me a long time ago. "Figures don't lie, but liars, figure." I like numbers because they are fixed, not ambiguous. But as I have come to realize, numbers can often be manipulated and presented in various ways that can often give a perception that is not very representative of reality. Numbers themselves are fixed but what they represent, how they are calculated, reached, or derived can cause the number to mislead others as to what the numbers really mean. Sometimes it may be difficult to realize it unless you pay attention and do a little research. I do not allege that anyone intentionally is trying to lie to the public or intends to mislead anyone. Others might make such claims. That is another conversation and not the intention of this book. I do admit that depending on one's personal agenda, he or she can present "data" or "scientific findings" in a way that could support different agendas. Some may intentionally use the term "science" or "scientific" to make their claims seem more credible, but one should verify what someone claims as science or scientific is really that and not just rhetoric. Me, I just want to point out to you the data, make you aware of ways that some may misunderstand, be misled, and give perspective so you can be aware, better informed, and reach your own conclusion. When I set out on this journey, I had many questions and I wanted to find the "honest answers." I want to emphasize to you how things are counted and how the "numbers" can be biased to inflate (or reduce) death counts from what they really may be.

One final thought. The number of weekly deaths from COVID-19 has come down considerably from the high of 16,350 reached on the week ending April 18, 2020. Last reported June 20, 2020 it was down to 481. I hope it will be zero soon and stay there, but realize that the number of cases diagnosed is rising, particularly in certain states so statistically the number of deaths may start to rise again, with the lag in time for the disease to progress and data to make it to the entities that report the official deaths. While many may be afraid of COVID-19 and wonder if this will ever end, I remain optimistic and try to look for the "silver lining" when possible.

- This country has been through many tough things and has always come through it. We survived the Spanish Flu in 1918-1919 that had a much higher Infection Fatality Rate of 10% when this one seems to have one around 1.0-1.5%. It may turn out to be much lower than this i.e. 50% lower or more. During 1918-1919, there was no lockdown of businesses as there were in 2020, and they did not have the knowledge or resources that we have today.

- We may have lower infection rates and deaths from other illnesses as a result from what the public is doing. Cases of influenza A & B along with other respiratory infections may be reduced in the future because of better hygiene practices i.e. hand washing, face covering, "coughing into elbow," disinfecting, etc. Hepatitis A and other infectious diseases may be reduced. Anecdotal reports of fewer deaths related to motor vehicle collisions during shelter in place are already being made.

- We have already learned a lot about this SARS-CoV-2 and will continue to do so.
  - We know certain things that may help prevent the spread and our population has done a good job doing its part i.e. masks, social distancing, hand washing
  - Quarantining or sheltering those at most risk i.e. elderly, immunocompromised, those with underlying health conditions (comorbidities)
  - The chances of surviving an infection from SARS-CoV-2 (COVID-19) seems to already be improving. Treatments are being discovered, studies are being conducted and great efforts for vaccines are being undertaken.
  - Two medications already approved for other uses, dexamethasone, and hydroxychloroquine, have been used in studies that are encouraging. The medications may help reduce the mortality of severely ill and/or hospitalized patients.
- While no one wants the virus to spread, the silver lining is that its spread may be what ultimately gets our country, and others around the globe, out of this mess. Unless immunity can be developed, we will always be "in danger" of its spread. Two ways for immunity to develop are effective vaccines and previous infections, and the development of effective antibodies to the virus (neutralizing antibodies). Some call this herd immunity. In simple terms, if everyone else (the herd) is immune, there is protection to you, even if you are not immune because "no one" will spread it to you. It is believed that 50-70% of the population would need to have immunity (effective or neutralizing antibodies to SARS-CoV-2) to achieve herd immunity and impede the spread of the virus, whether by vaccine or infection. FYI.

The more contagious a virus, the higher the percentage of a population with immunity must be to provide protection to those who are not immune.

- No one is advocating for anyone to go out and intentionally catch the illness, but as more people do become infected, those who recover seem to develop antibodies to the SARS-CoV-2 virus that causes COVID-19. We do not know for certain, if these antibodies will protect us, but we are not sure it will not protect us either. If I had to make an educated guess based on my understanding of the human immune system and past viruses including the closely related SARS-CoV-1 of 2002-2003, it is reasonable to say that there is a reasonable chance that those who catch SARS-CoV-2 and recover will likely develop antibodies to it, may become immune, and not spread it.[cxli]

- No guarantee but mentioning the optimistic view. Unless there is an effective vaccine that prevents it, or a medication that cures it once contracted, there are not too many other options. Of course, we could shut down the economy, keep people in lockdown and destroy or change our way of life forever, or until the day we have a cure or an effective vaccine. I am not sure too many people want to do that or whether this is a realistic option, particularly when one considers the human suffering and financial costs of a lockdown. This will be discussed in much greater detail in the next book in this series (*Lockdown 2020: Consequences & Perspective*)

I hope this book, *COVID-19 Lockdown: Unreported Truths & Perspective,* has been informative to you and helps you better understand the current "pandemic." Hopefully, this can help you better understand what others are saying and even know when others are not saying things that make sense or that may be communicating things that are not supported by the data.

Data that you can look up and verify. Certainly, I hope this helps lessen some of the fear and panic that I am concerned exists that is not necessary and does not help matters. There is no reason to scare people. Some may believe this is the only way to get, convince or force people to do what you want. Perhaps? Personally, I believe in informing people. Give them the appropriate, accurate and complete (as much as possible or needed) to make informed decisions. Trust people to do what is right and what is best for them. Hold them accountable for their actions. I believe people should respect one another and not try to harm, intimidate, or scare others, and we will all be much better off individually, and as a country.

In my upcoming book, *Lockdown 2020: Consequences & Perspective*, I will discuss the consequences of the lockdown particularly focusing on all of the human suffering and deaths that can be caused as a result of the "policy" and/or decision of causing so many to suddenly become unemployed, preventing people from earning a living and the human health and suffering consequences that has and can result from it. Many may say the consequences are much worse than what COVID-19 caused, much worse. I will point out miscues that were made and discuss what we have learned and how we can help prevent another pandemic from happening or at least, mitigating the damage, economic and human suffering that might occur. Rest assured; I am confident that America will get through this. We always seem to make it through tough times and come out stronger than before. Stay safe, stay informed, ask many questions, practice good hygiene, protect yourself and others, use good judgment, apply common sense, and live a healthy life. Until we connect again...

[i] Scher, Isaac. July 1, 2020. < https://www.msn.com/en-us/news/world/the-first-covid-19-case-originated-on-november-17-according-to-chinese-officials-searching-for-patient-zero/ar-BB119fWJ>

[ii] Westcott, Ben. June 23, 2020. < https://www.cnn.com/2019/06/02/asia/tiananmen-square-june-1989-intl/index.html>

[iii] Kelly, Jack. June 23, 2020. < https://www.forbes.com/sites/jackkelly/2020/03/05/china-moves-uyghur-muslims-into-forced-labor-factories/#164d7bf244e5>

[iv] Kelly, Jack. June 23, 2020. < https://www.forbes.com/sites/jackkelly/2020/03/05/china-moves-uyghur-muslims-into-forced-labor-factories/#164d7bf244e5>

[v] Su, Alice. June 24, 2020. <https://www.latimes.com/world-nation/story/2020-02-06/coronavirus-china-xi-li-wenliang>

[vi] Schumaker, Erin. June 23, 2020. < https://abcnews.go.com/Health/1st-confirmed-case-coronavirus-reported-washington-state-cdc/story?id=68430795>

[vii] McNamara, Audrey. July 1, 2020. < https://www.cbsnews.com/news/coronavirus-centers-for-disease-control-first-case-united-states/>

[viii] CDC. July 1, 2020. < https://www.cdc.gov/media/releases/2020/s0229-COVID-19-first-death.html>

[ix] Ballotpedia. June 23, 2020. <https://ballotpedia.org/Status_of_lockdown_and_stay-at-home_orders_in_response_to_the_coronavirus_(COVID-19)_pandemic,_2020>

[x] Timeanddate.com. June 23, 2020. <https://www.timeanddate.com/holidays/us/lockdown-day-1>

[xi] Santhanam, Laura. July 1, 2020. < https://www.pbs.org/newshour/economy/3-charts-reveal-how-the-covid-19-unemployment-crisis-isnt-over>

[xii] Marium-Webster.com. June 23, 2020. <https://www.merriam-webster.com/dictionary/coronavirus>

[xiii] Abcdust.net. July 1, 2020. < https://abcdust.net/how-large-is-a-corona-virus-virion-compared-to-the-mp10-2-5/>

[xiv] Lesney, Mark. June 21, 2020. <https://www.medscape.com/viewarticle/925710>

xv Wikipedia.org. June 24, 2020. <https://en.wikipedia.org/wiki/2002–2004_SARS_outbreak>

xvi News-medical.net. June 24, 2020. <https://www.news-medical.net/health/Origin-of-Lyme-Disease.aspx>

xvii Lowry, Rich. June 21, 2020. <https://nypost.com/2020/03/09/its-not-racist-to-call-it-the-wuhan-virus/>

xviii Lowry, Rich. June 21, 2020. <https://nypost.com/2020/03/09/its-not-racist-to-call-it-the-wuhan-virus/>

xix Lowry, Rich. June 21, 2020. <https://nypost.com/2020/03/09/its-not-racist-to-call-it-the-wuhan-virus/>

xx Lowry, Rich. June 21, 2020. <https://nypost.com/2020/03/09/its-not-racist-to-call-it-the-wuhan-virus/>

xxi Elci, Lee. June 21, 2020. <https://www.theday.com/article/20200318/OP04/200319395>

xxii World Health Organization. June 25, 2020. < https://www.who.int/ith/diseases/sars/en/>

xxiii Center for Disease Control and Prevention. June 25, 2020. < https://www.cdc.gov/coronavirus/2019-ncov/prevent-getting-sick/how-covid-spreads.html>

xxiv Givas, Nick. June 25, 2020. < https://www.foxnews.com/world/world-health-organization-january-tweet-china-human-transmission-coronavirus>

xxv Givas, Nick. June 25, 2020. < https://www.foxnews.com/world/world-health-organization-january-tweet-china-human-transmission-coronavirus>

xxvi WebMD. June 25, 2020. <https://www.webmd.com/lung/coronavirus-transmission-overview#1>

xxvii CDC. June 28, 2020. < https://www.cdc.gov/coronavirus/2019-ncov/need-extra-precautions/people-at-increased-risk.html?CDC_AA_refVal=https%3A%2F%2Fwww.cdc.gov%2Fcoronavirus%2F2019-ncov%2Fneed-extra-precautions%2Fpeople-at-higher-risk.html>

xxviii 3M. July 1, 2020. < https://workersafety.3m.com/differences-disposable-respirators-surgical-masks/#:~:text=The%20two%20types%20also%20fit%20differently%2C%20with%20respirators,certain%20regulatory%20standards%20also%20differ%20between%20the%20two.>

xxix CDC. July 1, 2020. <https://www.cdc.gov/tb/webcourses/course/chapter7/7_infection_c

ontrol_7_infection_control_program_respirators_vs._surgical_masks.
html>

[xxx] Occupational Safety and Health Administration. July 1, 2020. <
https://www.osha.gov/video/respiratory_protection/resptypes_transc
ript.html#:~:text=The%20first%20part%20of%20the%20filter%27s%20
classification%20uses,%22P%22%20means%20strongly%20resistant%
20to%20oil%2C%20or%20oil-Proof.>

[xxxi] Occupational Safety and Health Administration. July 1, 2020. <
https://www.osha.gov/video/respiratory_protection/resptypes_transc
ript.html#:~:text=The%20first%20part%20of%20the%20filter%27s%20
classification%20uses,%22P%22%20means%20strongly%20resistant%
20to%20oil%2C%20or%20oil-Proof.>

[xxxii] Canadian Centre for Occupational Health and Safety. July 1, 2020.
<https://www.ccohs.ca/oshanswers/prevention/ppe/surgical_mask.ht
ml>

[xxxiii] Virginia Polytechnic Institute and State University. July 1, 2020. <
https://www.ehss.vt.edu/uploaded_docs/201402031829220.NRP%20
Designations.pdf>

[xxxiv] Litke, Eric. July 1, 2020. <
https://www.usatoday.com/story/news/factcheck/2020/06/11/fact-
check-n-95-filters-not-too-large-stop-covid-19-
particles/5343537002/>

[xxxv] Abcdust.net. July 1, 2020. < https://abcdust.net/how-large-is-a-
corona-virus-virion-compared-to-the-mp10-2-5/>

[xxxvi] Litke, Eric. July 1, 2020. <
https://www.usatoday.com/story/news/factcheck/2020/06/11/fact-
check-n-95-filters-not-too-large-stop-covid-19-
particles/5343537002/>

[xxxvii] Litke, Eric. July 1, 2020. <
https://www.usatoday.com/story/news/factcheck/2020/06/11/fact-
check-n-95-filters-not-too-large-stop-covid-19-
particles/5343537002/>

[xxxviii] Litke, Eric. July 1, 2020. <
https://www.usatoday.com/story/news/factcheck/2020/06/11/fact-
check-n-95-filters-not-too-large-stop-covid-19-
particles/5343537002/>

[xxxix] Globalsecurity.com. June 25, 2020. <
https://www.globalsecurity.org/security/ops/hsc-scen-3_flu-
pandemic-
deaths.htm#:~:text=During%20a%20typical%20year%20in%20the%20

United%20States%2C,for%20influenza%20lead%20to%20fatal%20outc
ome%20in%20adults.>

[xl] Jones, Stephen, Moyer, Tyler. June 21, 2020.
<https://www.bakersfieldnow.com/news/local/accelerated-urgent-
care-provides-statistical-update-on-covid-19>

[xli] Wright, Anthony. June.
<https://www.turnto23.com/news/coronavirus/watch-controversial-
press-conference-held-by-two-bakersfield-doctors-that-was-pulled-
down-by-youtube>

[xlii] Wright, Anthony. June.
<https://www.turnto23.com/news/coronavirus/watch-controversial-
press-conference-held-by-two-bakersfield-doctors-that-was-pulled-
down-by-youtube>

[xliii] Jones, Stephen, Moyer, Tyler. June 21, 2020.
<https://www.bakersfieldnow.com/news/local/accelerated-urgent-
care-provides-statistical-update-on-covid-19>

[xliv] Jones, Stephen, Moyer, Tyler. June 21, 2020.
<https://www.bakersfieldnow.com/news/local/accelerated-urgent-
care-provides-statistical-update-on-covid-19>

[xlv] Jones, Stephen, Moyer, Tyler. June 21, 2020.
<https://www.bakersfieldnow.com/news/local/accelerated-urgent-
care-provides-statistical-update-on-covid-19>

[xlvi] Palca, Joe. June 25, 2020.
<https://www.npr.org/sections/coronavirus-live-
updates/2020/06/15/877498151/fda-withdraws-emergency-use-
authorization-for-hydroxychloroquine>

[xlvii] Yahoo.com. June 25, 2020. <https://news.yahoo.com/zinc-
hydroxychloroquine-found-effective-covid-19-patients-study-
215732283.html>

[xlviii] Palca, Joe. June 25, 2020.
<https://www.npr.org/sections/coronavirus-live-
updates/2020/06/15/877498151/fda-withdraws-emergency-use-
authorization-for-hydroxychloroquine>

[xlix] Palca, Joe. June 25, 2020.
<https://www.npr.org/sections/coronavirus-live-
updates/2020/06/15/877498151/fda-withdraws-emergency-use-
authorization-for-hydroxychloroquine>

[l] EraofLight.com. June 25, 2020.
<https://eraoflight.com/2020/04/11/french-study-of-1000-patients-
see-98-success-rate-with-hydroxychloroquine-azithromycin-regimen/>

[li] Dall, Chris. June 25, 2020. Cidrap.umn.edu/news-perspective/2020/05/studies-find-further-lack-covid-benefit-hydroxychloroquine>

[lii] Edwards, Erika. June 25, 2020. <https://www.nbcnews.com/health/health-news/lancet-retracts-large-study-hydroxychloroquine-n1225091>

[liii] Edwards, Erika. June 25, 2020. <https://www.nbcnews.com/health/health-news/lancet-retracts-large-study-hydroxychloroquine-n1225091>

[liv] CBS News. June 25, 2020. <<https://www.cbsnews.com/news/dexamethasone-coronavirus-death-risk-severe-cases-study/>

[lv] Edwards, Erika. June 25, 2020. <https://www.nbcnews.com/health/health-news/lancet-retracts-large-study-hydroxychloroquine-n1225091>

[lvi] Edwards, Erika. June 25, 2020. <https://www.nbcnews.com/health/health-news/lancet-retracts-large-study-hydroxychloroquine-n1225091>

[lvii] Henry Ford Health System. July 3, 2020. < https://www.henryford.com/news/2020/07/hydro-treatment-study>

[lviii] Palca, Joe. June 25, 2020. <https://www.npr.org/sections/coronavirus-live-updates/2020/06/15/877498151/fda-withdraws-emergency-use-authorization-for-hydroxychloroquine>

[lix] National Institute of Health. June 25, 2020. <https://www.covid19treatmentguidelines.nih.gov/antiviral-therapy/remdesivir/>

[lx] Reuters. June 25, 2020. <https://reuters.com/article/us-health-coronavirus-gilead-europe-idUSKBN23W1ZH>

[lxi] Marchione, Marilynn. June 25, 2020. <https://www.usatoday.com/story/news/health/2020/06/16/conoavirus-drug-steroid-dexamethasone-reduce-covid-deaths/3197420001/>

[lxii] CBS News. June 25, 2020. <<https://www.cbsnews.com/news/dexamethasone-coronavirus-death-risk-severe-cases-study/>

[lxiii] Drugs.com. June 25, 2020. < https://www.drugs.com/medical-answers/tamiflu-work-covid-19-3537049/>

[lxiv] Drugs.com. June 25, 2020. < https://www.drugs.com/medical-answers/tamiflu-work-covid-19-3537049/>

[lxv] Marchione, Marilynn. June 25, 2020.
<https://www.usatoday.com/story/news/health/2020/06/16/conoavi
rus-drug-steroid-dexamethasone-reduce-covid-deaths/3197420001/>
[lxvi] CBS News. June 25, 2020.
<<https://www.cbsnews.com/news/dexamethasone-coronavirus-
death-risk-severe-cases-study/>
[lxvii] Rivas, Kayla. June 25, 2020.
<https://www.foxnews.com/health/preliminary-dexamethasone-data-
published-life-saving-coronavirus-drug>
[lxviii] Marchione, Marilynn. June 25, 2020.
<https://www.usatoday.com/story/news/health/2020/06/16/conoavi
rus-drug-steroid-dexamethasone-reduce-covid-deaths/3197420001/>
[lxix] CBS News. June 25, 2020.
<<https://www.cbsnews.com/news/dexamethasone-coronavirus-
death-risk-severe-cases-study/>
[lxx] CBS News. June 25, 2020.
<<https://www.cbsnews.com/news/dexamethasone-coronavirus-
death-risk-severe-cases-study/>
[lxxi] Marchione, Marilynn. June 25, 2020.
<https://www.usatoday.com/story/news/health/2020/06/16/conoavi
rus-drug-steroid-dexamethasone-reduce-covid-deaths/3197420001/>
[lxxii] Rivas, Kayla. June 25, 2020.
<https://www.foxnews.com/health/preliminary-dexamethasone-data-
published-life-saving-coronavirus-drug>
[lxxiii] Marchione, Marilynn. June 25, 2020.
<https://www.usatoday.com/story/news/health/2020/06/16/conoavi
rus-drug-steroid-dexamethasone-reduce-covid-deaths/3197420001/>
[lxxiv] Columbia University Irving Medical Center. June 25, 2020. <
https://www.cuimc.columbia.edu/news/thrombosis-emerges-
significant-risk-covid-19-patients>
[lxxv] Columbia University Irving Medical Center. June 25, 2020.
<https://www.cuimc.columbia.edu/news/thrombosis-emerges-
significant-risk-covid-19-patients>
[lxxvi] Columbia University Irving Medical Center. June 25, 2020.
<https://www.cuimc.columbia.edu/news/thrombosis-emerges-
significant-risk-covid-19-patients>
[lxxvii] Worldometers.info. June 21, 2020.
<https://www.worldometers.info/coronavirus/coronavirus-death-
rate/#who-03-03-20>
[lxxviii] CDC. June 21, 2020.
<https://www.cdc.gov/nchs/nvss/vsrr/covid19/excess_deaths.htm>

[lxxix] CDC. June 21, 2020. <
https://www.cdc.gov/nchs/nvss/vsrr/covid19/excess_deaths.htm>
[lxxx] Wikipedia. June 29, 2020. <
https://en.wikipedia.org/wiki/Mortality_rate>
[lxxxi] Imperial College London. June 21, 2020.
<https://imperial,ac.uk/mrc-global-infectious-disease-analysis/covid-19/report-12-global-impact-covid-19/>
[lxxxii] Imperial College London. June 21, 2020.
<https://imperial,ac.uk/mrc-global-infectious-disease-analysis/covid-19/report-12-global-impact-covid-19/>
[lxxxiii] Shefrin, Hersh. June 27, 2020. <
https://www.forbes.com/sites/hershshefrin/2020/04/18/what-makes-the-covid-19-mortality-forecasts-upon-which-the-white-house-relies-seem-so-low/#18eb1ca72f70>
[lxxxiv] Shefrin, Hersh. June 27, 2020. <
https://www.forbes.com/sites/hershshefrin/2020/04/18/what-makes-the-covid-19-mortality-forecasts-upon-which-the-white-house-relies-seem-so-low/#18eb1ca72f70>
[lxxxv] CDC. June 21, 2020. <https://www.cdc.gov/flu/pandemic-resources/1918-pandemic-h1n1.html>
[lxxxvi] Bing. July 4, 2020. <
https://www.bing.com/search?q=causes+of+the+common+cold&form=EDGEAR&qs=AS&cvid=46b6b017d73c47828a403ef1d8e7c6fe&cc=US&setlang=en-US&plvar=0&PC=HCTS>
[lxxxvii] Worldometers.info. June 27, 2020. <
https://www.worldometers.info/world-population/>
[lxxxviii] United States Census Bureau. June 27, 2020.
<https://www.census.gov/popclock/>
[lxxxix] Askthe odds.com. July 4, 2020. <
http://www.asktheodds.com/death/car-crash-odds/>
[xc] CDC. July 4, 2020. <
https://www.cdc.gov/drugoverdose/data/statedeaths.html>
[xci] Federal Drug Administration. June 27, 2020.
<https://www.fda.gov/emergency-preparedness-and-response/mcm-legal-regulatory-and-policy-framework/emergency-use-authorization>
[xcii] Federal Drug Administration. June 27, 2020.
<https://www.fda.gov/emergency-preparedness-and-response/mcm-legal-regulatory-and-policy-framework/emergency-use-authorization>
[xciii] Associated Press. June 21, 2020.
<https://www.modernhealthcare.com/technology/accuracy-covid-19-tests-still-largely-unknown>

[xcivxciv] Associated Press. June 21, 2020.
<https://www.modernhealthcare.com/technology/accuracy-covid-19-tests-still-largely-unknown>

[xcv] CDC. June 27. 2020. <https://www.cdc.gov/coronavirus/2019-ncov/downloads/OASH-COVID-19-guidance-testing-platforms.pdf>

[xcvi] Zhao, Yongxi, Chen,Feng, Li, Qian, Wang, Lihua, Fan, Chunhai. June 27, 2020. <https://pubs.acs.org/doi/10.1021/acs.chemrev.5b00428>

[xcvii] Zhao, Yongxi, Chen,Feng, Li, Qian, Wang, Lihua, Fan, Chunhai. June 27, 2020. <https://pubs.acs.org/doi/10.1021/acs.chemrev.5b00428>

[xcviii] CDC. June 27. 2020. <https://www.cdc.gov/coronavirus/2019-ncov/downloads/OASH-COVID-19-guidance-testing-platforms.pdf>

[xcix] Plumbo, Ginger. June 27, 2020.
<https://www.newsnetwork.mayoclinic.org/discussion/mayo-clinic-launches-neutralizing-antibody-test-to-advance-covid-19-therapies/#>

[c] Plumbo, Ginger. June 27, 2020.
<https://www.newsnetwork.mayoclinic.org/discussion/mayo-clinic-launches-neutralizing-antibody-test-to-advance-covid-19-therapies/#>

[ci] Lin, Qingging, Zhu, Li, Ni, Zuowei, Meng, Haito, You, Liangshun. June 27, 2020.
<https://www.ncbi.nlm.nih.gov/pmc/articles/PMC7141458/>

[cii] Lin, Qingging, Zhu, Li, Ni, Zuowei, Meng, Haito, You, Liangshun. June 27, 2020.
<https://www.ncbi.nlm.nih.gov/pmc/articles/PMC7141458/>

[ciii] Lin, Qingging, Zhu, Li, Ni, Zuowei, Meng, Haito, You, Liangshun. June 27, 2020.
<https://www.ncbi.nlm.nih.gov/pmc/articles/PMC7141458/>

[civ] Dunn, Lauren. June 21, 2020.
<https://www.nbcnews.com/health/health-news/questions-about-covid-19-test-accuracy-raised-across-testing-spectrum-n1214981>

[cv] Accesalabs.com. June 27, 2020.
<https://support.accesalabs.com/article/65-what-does-sensitivity-mean-what-does-specificity-mean>

[cvi] Associated Press. June 21, 2020.
<https://www.modernhealthcare.com/technology/accuracy-covid-19-tests-still-largely-unknown>

[cvii] Associated Press. June 21, 2020.
<https://www.modernhealthcare.com/technology/accuracy-covid-19-tests-still-largely-unknown>

[cviii] Associated Press. June 21, 2020.
<https://www.modernhealthcare.com/technology/accuracy-covid-19-tests-still-largely-unknown>

[cix] Associated Press. June 21, 2020.
<https://www.modernhealthcare.com/technology/accuracy-covid-19-tests-still-largely-unknown>
[cx] Associated Press. June 21, 2020.
<https://www.modernhealthcare.com/technology/accuracy-covid-19-tests-still-largely-unknown>
[cxi] Associated Press. June 21, 2020.
<https://www.modernhealthcare.com/technology/accuracy-covid-19-tests-still-largely-unknown>
[cxii] Dunn, Lauren. June 21, 2020.
<https://www.nbcnews.com/health/health-news/questions-about-covid-19-test-accuracy-raised-across-testing-spectrum-n1214981>
[cxiii] Associated Press. June 21, 2020.
<https://www.modernhealthcare.com/technology/accuracy-covid-19-tests-still-largely-unknown>
[cxiv] Dunn, Lauren. June 21, 2020.
<https://www.nbcnews.com/health/health-news/questions-about-covid-19-test-accuracy-raised-across-testing-spectrum-n1214981>
[cxv] Dunn, Lauren. June 21, 2020.
<https://www.nbcnews.com/health/health-news/questions-about-covid-19-test-accuracy-raised-across-testing-spectrum-n1214981>
[cxvi] Dunn, Lauren. June 21, 2020.
<https://www.nbcnews.com/health/health-news/questions-about-covid-19-test-accuracy-raised-across-testing-spectrum-n1214981>
[cxvii] Johns Hopkins University. June 28, 2020.
<https://www.coronavirus.jhu.edu/data/mortality>
[cxviii] CDC. June 28, 2020. <https://www.cdc.gov/coronavirus/2019-ncov/cases-updates/cases-in-us.html>
[cxix] CDC. June 28, 2020. <https://www.cdc.gov/coronavirus/2019-ncov/cases-updates/cases-in-us.html>
[cxx] CDC. June 29, 2020. <https://www.cdc.gov/NCHS/Provisional-COVID-19-Death-Counts-by-Sex-Age-and-S/9bhg-hcku>
[cxxi] CDC. June 29, 2020. <https://www.cdc.gov/NCHS/Provisional-COVID-19-Death-Counts-by-Sex-Age-and-S/9bhg-hcku>
[cxxiicxxii] CDC. July 4, 2020. <
https://www.cdc.gov/flu/about/burden/index.html>
[cxxiii] Romo, Vanessa. May 19, 2020. <
https://www.opb.org/news/article/npr-for-most-states-at-least-a-third-of-covid-19-deaths-are-in-long-term-care-facilities/>
[cxxiv] CDC. June 29, 2020. <https://www.cdc.gov/nchs/fastats/leading-causes-of-death.htm>

cxxv National Center for Health Statistics. June 29, 2020.
<https://www.cdc.gov/nchs/data/nvsr/nvsr68/nvsr68_09-508.pdf>
cxxvi PopulationPyramid.net. June 29, 2020. <
https://www.populationpyramid.net/united-states-of-america/2017/>
cxxvii National Center for Health Statistics. June 29, 2020.
<https://www.cdc.gov/nchs/data/nvsr/nvsr68/nvsr68_09-508.pdf>
cxxviii Gallagher, Grant M. July 4, 2020. <
https://www.contagionlive.com/news/persontoperson-transmission-
confirmed-in-novel-coronavirus-outbreak>
cxxixcxxix National Center for Health Statistics. June 29, 2020.
<https://www.cdc.gov/nchs/nvss/vsrr/covid19/index.htm>
cxxx Weiss, Jonathan. July 3, 2020. <
https://www.medicaldaily.com/half-men-over-60-have-prostate-
cancer-most-die-other-causes-247635>
cxxxi CDC. June 28, 2020.
<https://www.cdc.gov/nchs/data/nvss/coronavirus/Understanding-
COVID-19-Provisional-Death-Counts.pdf>
cxxxii CDC. June 28, 2020.
<https://www.cdc.gov/nchs/data/nvss/coronavirus/Understanding-
COVID-19-Provisional-Death-Counts.pdf>
cxxxiii CDC. June 21, 2020. <
https://www.cdc.gov/nchs/nvss/vsrr/covid19/excess_deaths.htm>
cxxxiv CDC. June 21, 2020. <
https://www.cdc.gov/nchs/nvss/vsrr/covid19/excess_deaths.htm>
cxxxv CDC. June 21, 2020. <
https://www.cdc.gov/nchs/nvss/vsrr/covid19/excess_deaths.htm>
cxxxvi BBC. June 28, 2020. <https://www.bbc.com/news/world-us-
canada-52303739>
cxxxvii BBC. June 28, 2020. <https://www.bbc.com/news/world-us-
canada-52303739>
cxxxviii BBC. June 28, 2020. <https://www.bbc.com/news/world-us-
canada-52303739>
cxxxix Worldometers.info. June 21, 2020.
<https://www.worldometers.info/coronavirus/coronavirus-death-
rate/#who-03-03-20>
cxl Worldometers.info. June 21, 2020.
<https://www.worldometers.info/coronavirus/coronavirus-death-
rate/#who-03-03-20>
cxli Lin, Qingging, Zhu, Li, Ni, Zuowei, Meng, Haito, You, Liangshun. June
27, 2020.
<https://www.ncbi.nlm.nih.gov/pmc/articles/PMC7141458/>

www.ingramcontent.com/pod-product-compliance
Lightning Source LLC
Chambersburg PA
CBHW022119280326
41933CB00007B/453